The Medical Student's Guide to Top Board Scores

P. Thomas Rogers, M.D.

Also by this author:

Spanish for Health Care Professionals
A user friendly introduction to medical Spanish.
Cassette & Guide
© 1988

Medical Spanish for Pediatrics
A concise, systematic pocket booklet that parallels the pediatric history and physical examination.
© 1991

For ordering information please call 312/996-4493

Published in the United States
by Innovative Publishing & Graphics, Inc., Chicago.

Printed in the United States of America
First Edition

ISBN 0-9632231-0-0

ACKNOWLEDGEMENTS

I would like to express my appreciation to the many people who either directly or indirectly helped with this book including: Diana Krug, Shi Young, Kevin Koy, Rolando Toyos, Dr. William Wallace, Dr. David Toovy, Dr. Chuck Kinder, Dr. Sanjay RevanKar, Frank Agatucci, Dr. Tamara Wyse, Dr. Truman Anderson, Frank Sparks, Barbara Karklins, Jaime Rivas, Marsha Davis, Debra Baines, Neil Bhattarychya, Peggy Wheeler, Dr. Jorge Girotti, Nellie Clark, Tom Betlej, Dr. Bernadette Gochiuco, Dr. Ike Kim, Jeanie An, Paul DeFrino, Dr. Kevin Hannon and Susie Rogers-Hannon, Mark Rogers, Michelle Zafrani, Michael Rogers Jr., Sandy Vega, Phil Levin, all of the medical students at the University of Illinois, and of course most of all my parents, Dr. Michael and Olga Rogers.

Contents

FOREWORD

I was honored when Dr. P. Thomas Rogers asked me to write the foreword of his book on studying for the National Boards exam. As of the Spring of 1991 a new examination called United States Medical Licensure Examination was initiated by the National Board of Medical Examiners. This exam was designed to test the medical students understanding of basic science principles with many questions requiring assessment of clinical situations, interpretation of tabular material and identification of gross and microscopic specimens.

Although basic science discoveries form the foundation for modern health care, it is often difficult to initially see the correlations between laboratory findings and pragmatic usefulness at the clinical bedside. One of the strong points of this book is that it emphasizes clinical aspects of basic science material. Today, more than ever there is a great need for cross-fertilization between the basic scientist and the clinical scientist and too few opportunities are available for this exchange. However, a continued interaction is especially important as the competition for limited funds becomes more critical and as medicine advances into the twenty first century.

With regards to the medical licensure examination we appreciate the fact that in the past, National Boards has never been shown to be a good predictor of clinical competence, yet we are also aware of the reality of its tremendous impact in the residency selection process. We therefore believe that a well conceived preparation for the National Boards must be part of a student's effort while in medical school. It is for that reason Dr. Rogers has written this book.

I have known Dr. Rogers ever since he began medical school. He came from Stanford University where he had graduated with distinction in biology. He is an outstanding student as represented by his first percentile score on the National Boards part I exam. Currently, he is completing his clinical internship as part of his residency in diagnostic imaging at Northwestern University Medical School. While in medical school he worked as a teaching assistant or tutor for most of the basic science courses. His mnemonics and study strategies were considered extremely helpful by the medical students who encouraged him to collect his methods into a book. This is the book. I believe that this text will be a valuable instrument for students preparing for part I of the U.S. Medical Licensure Examination.

William Wallace PhD
Dean of Academic Student Affairs
University of Illinois Medical School

PREFACE

The purpose of *The Medical Student's Guide to Top Board Scores* (MSGTBS) is to help you score high on your school exams and the national boards medical licensing examination. This book provides you with specific strategic approaches for each of the 7 sections on the part I exam as well as a listing of the most highly recommended textbooks as judged by medical students who all scored in the top 5% on this exam. The section on national boards is followed by an extensive collection of mnemonics.

Mnemonics facilitate rapid learning and long term memory. These mnemonics cover essential parts of general medical knowledge and will be helpful to you throughout your career. Mnemonics have been used successfully for each of the basic sciences, but are most effective for anatomy, biochemistry and pathology. The mnemonics for the history and physical and the mental status exam provide a frame of reference that will help you to make the transition from classroom to clinical medicine.

MSGTBS also has several microbiology mnemonics which are incorporated into the section entitled "Microbiology Synopsis" which is a concise overview of clinical microbiology. It represents a distillation of the most important information from a wide variety of sources and places strong emphasis on classification and word association which are key concepts for learning microbiology. It has a user friendly outline format that quickly gives you the big picture and facilitates more efficient studying.

Speaking of which, MSGTBS contains an entire section devoted to study methods. The workload in medical school is a lot heavier than it was in college and you will have to fine tune your study habits to keep up with it. Increased efficiency will pay off in terms of better grades and more time left over for other things in life. In terms of study skills, the most important concept is that to be a successful student you have to develop some type of memory system for long term retention.

It is useful to think of national boards medical licensing exam part I as the final exam for the basic science material covered during the first two years of medical school. Although this test is a big time pain in the neck you should prepare for it as well as you can. Part I board scores are the primary screening device used by residency programs in all fields, but especially in the more competitive fields such as ophthalmology, radiology, orthopedics, ENT and dermatology.

I hope that this book helps you to reach your academic goals. Please send me any suggestions or criticisms you have which might improve this book. If you know of any mnemonics which would be beneficial to other students please send them in. Please include the authors name so that credit can be given, or write author not known (ANK). Finally, regardless of your board scores don't ever forget that in the eyes of your patients and your peers the characteristics of hardwork, common sense, kindness and dedication to the patient are much, much more important.

P. Thomas Rogers M. D.

Chapter 1
Study Strategies

STUDY STRATEGIES

I. INTRODUCTION

As recently as 30 years ago medical knowledge was taught mostly from large texts written in prose with few pictures, diagrams, or subtitles. These texts were subsequently improved by the addition of more pictures and diagrams, as well as shorter, more concise "baby versions" of the larger books. Soon afterwards came an outpouring of question books. The initial primitive questions books were improved by the selection of better questions, more detailed answers and a format that paralleled the NB exam.

Nowadays, there are so many different shapes and sizes of books for every topic that it is difficult to choose which one is right for you (see section on "How to select a book"). The best of the newer texts usually have more sophisticated schematic diagrams, more subtitles, more pictures and so on.

Another recent addition to the medical student's arsenal, in the battle for knowledge, is the mnemonic. Actually mnemonics have been around for a long time and were often passed by word of mouth from generation to generation of students. However, it is only recently that they have become an accepted part of textbooks.

The Medical Student's Guide to Top Board Scores provides you with mnemonics (Mn's) that cover essential parts of medical knowledge. Mn's provide a shelf/framework onto which new items can be added. They facilitate recall because the material is organized into a user friendly, familiar format, and the details can be derived from the basic concepts. Mn's are just one of the several memory systems that will be discussed.

Without a memory system, new information just gets haphazardly piled onto the old stuff which is prone to being gradually forgotten. This approach is frustrating and often leads to the "in one ear and out the other syndrome". What's the use of learning something if you can't remember it, or at least find it quickly?

Most of the Mn's in this book were written by the author. For the other Mn's, every attempt has been made to give credit to the original author. This is not always possible since many were learned via anonymous conversations among medical students. The abbreviation ANK is placed next to the title for the Mn's where the Author is Not Known. If you are aware of any authors who deserve credit for a Mn, please write to us and we will make sure credit is given in future editions, if this book reaches that point.

II. MOTIVATION

Study time is more productive and more enjoyable when you are motivated. The following information and study strategies will help you to stay motivated.

1. **Good grades**: Good grades will help you get a good residency position. This is especially important if you are considering going into orthopaedics, ophthalmology, radiology, dermatology, emergency medicine, neurosurgery, or other highly competitive fields.

2. **Knowledge**: Medical education builds on itself and most of what you learn as an M-1 will prepare you for M-2 topics and so on into the clinical years.

3. **Interest**: Try to stay/become interested in those subjects which are particularly dry. For example, you might think to

yourself, "maybe I will go into this or a related field." Most medical subjects are interesting and they are often more interrelated than is initially evident.

4. **Reward yourself**: After completing some work, reward yourself with your favorite meal, shopping, phone calls, exercise, or whatever.

III. When to Study

1. Study difficult topics when your brain is fresh, for example, in the morning or early evening. Later on, you can squeeze in your easier homework and busywork assignments.

2. Develop a routine to make sure you are getting enough study time. For example, you could wake up a little bit early and skim a copy of last year's notes before going to class. Later in the day, after lectures, you can change gears with an extracurricular activity before dinner. After dinner is a good time to study, although occasionally you may prefer to take a nap or watch your favorite t.v. show. In general, most students study a lot more in medical school than they did in college. As the year goes on, you will notice your "study endurance" actually increases. Conceptually, medical school subjects have about the same difficulty level as college courses, but the amount of material covered is much greater. Therefore you must learn to be efficient at studying and managing your time.

3. If you are having trouble getting enough study time, make a list of the distractions and try to minimize these.

IV. Where to Study

Anyplace that meets the basic requirements should be adequate:

1. Quiet
2. Minimal distractions
3. Music can be used to decrease outside distractions. In general, classical music such as Arcangelo Corelli, Bach, Handel, and Vivaldi works better than heavy metal.

V. What to Study

1. The lecture material is most important, since this is what you will be tested on.
2. Try to select the best books (See section on "How to Select a Book").
3. In general, it's better to study from relatively short books. You can always look up the rare, esoteric stuff in a large reference text or medical dictionary.
4. Do a lot of study questions, and, if possible, get a copy of the old tests. Quite often these will overlap considerably with the current exam.
5. Make it your goal to learn the material. If you learn the material and do the available study questions and question books, the grades will take care of themselves.

VI. How to Study

1. **Memory Systems:** The most important concept in this whole book is that to be a successful student, you have to develop some type of memory system for long term retention. The National Boards part I will test you on the subjects covered during the first and second medical school years. The coursework in medical school is not more difficult than it was in college. The main difference is that there is a ton more material covered with each class. Necessity is the mother of invention. So, develop a memory system for yourself. You can do this by studying the memory systems used by other persons and then adding your own twist to make it work for you. The term "memory system" is used here to mean any method of studying that facilitates long term retention. For example, Mn's are helpful for this purpose.

   Another useful approach is to make a single set of permanent, condensed notes for each topic. For example, NMS books and many other books are written in outline format. Therefore, they are already condensed. You can simply highlight the material that overlaps with lectures and then add additional notes in the margins.

   The margin spaces can also be used to summarize key concepts and for making your own Mn's. Make a note in the index when you add a topic that is not covered by the book. That way, you will always be able to find it quickly. Information is only useful if it is accessible.

   You can put other notes in the margins such as page numbers from lecture notes or other texts on the same topic. Thus, you will have a single set of permanent, condensed review notes with built in references. Note: Outline format books are often well suited for this, but any well written concise text with adequate subtitles will suffice.

2. **Condensed Notes:** As mentioned above, condensed notes are useful for quick review prior to exams. Highlighting, underlining, and making margin notes helps to personalize the text which facilitates long term recall and quick access.

3. **Organization:** Try to keep your information sources organized. This makes it easier to find information quickly, especially when going back to old notes while reviewing in preparation for the National Boards. Lecture notes can be put into binders and adhesive labels, paperclips, or "post-its" can be used to keep your place or to further subcategorize. Make your mind a file, not a pile. Try to stay reasonably caught up in your classes. You should know where you are in terms of how much material you have covered, and how much has been presented in lectures.

4. You may have heard of the link, peg and number rhyme systems of memory, These systems make it possible to remember long digit numbers and long lists of information. One useful little memory feat is the calendar trick, which enables you to determine the day of the week for any given date. You simply memorize the date for the 1st Sunday of each month, eg. 521-537-526-486 for 1992. Then when given a date you can calculate the corresponding day of the week, This can be useful for scheduling patient appointments among other things. By memorizing 12 numbers, you now know something about 365 numbers. Note: a similar concept is used in the mnemonic for glycolysis.

   These systems are especially useful when you don't have a pen or paper. When paper and pencil are available, it is much easier to just write stuff down. In my own experience of plowing through many books, workbooks and cassettes, I have found these memory techniques entertaining, but only minimally helpful for facilitating the ability to learn medical information. These systems are especially difficult to use with medical terms because so many words are so similar to each other. However, these systems do provide a powerful boost to memory for non-medical stuff, and reading several chapters or a book on the subject will probably sharpen your memory a little bit in all areas. The best book I've seen on the subject is, *Super Memory, Super Student* by Harry Lorayne.

5. **Question Books** Question books are extremely helpful. There is a somewhat limited number of relevant questions for each subject. On exams, you will have to answer questions.Therefore, up to a certain point of diminishing returns, the more practice questions you can answer, the better you will do on the exam.

6. **How to Use a Question Book**

   a. Go through the question book immediately after studying a subject.

   b. Look at the answer sheet and circle the correct answers. Do not waste time trying to "test" yourself. Circle the important stuff that you already know.

   c. Skim the questions and then read the answers one by one. Highlight or circle stuff you already know. If something new to you seems important, consider putting it into your condensed notes.

d. Basically, you are learning/memorizing the correct answers and then reading about the associated information.

e. Go through the question books again before school exams and the National Boards. Each time you will learn more and you will have seen these questions's several times before the National Boards.

VII. APPROACH TO CLASS / LECTURES

1. Go to class! Your class attendance should be almost 100%. One of the few exceptions is when the lecturer is really, really bad (eg. disorganized, uninformative). Then at least wake up, get out of bed and try to do something useful. For example, study the material that was to be covered in class.

2. There are several things you can do to get the most out of class. Read about the material in advance! For example, last years lecture notes, will make the lecture more understandable and will give you an edge in keeping up.

3. Sit near the front. Yes, it's true some of your classmates will mock you for this with phrases like "gunner" and "hardcore". However, if you are a nice person, they will soon forgive you, and you will eventually forgive them or at least pretend that you do. Anyway, it is in your best interest to sit up front where you can see better, hear better, and there are less distractions.

4. By going to lecture, you stay in touch with what's going on in your classes. You know exactly what was covered in

lecture, you receive handouts given out, and you are aware of any quizzes or homework for which you are responsible.

5. If your school has a co-op/classnotes system, then use it. These are lecture summary notes written by classmates for their classmates. Try to get a copy of last year's as well as this year's. That way, you can stay up to date and you will have at least one set of alternate notes in case any issue is missing or poorly written.

VIII. NOTETAKING

1. The main purpose of taking notes is to summarize the key points from lectures. Write neatly or print so that the notes will be legible for review.

2. Put a number or dash in the left margin for each item/concept as you write it down. Then when you review the notes, just check off each item number as you process it.

3. Use lots of abbreviations. This will increase your speed, so you can keep up with the lecturer.

4. Buy a 4-color pen. These are great for graphs, diagrams, and adding emphasis. For example, red can represent arteries, blue for veins, green for lymphatics, and black for nerves.

5. If given a handout, make notes in the margins.

6. Review your notes the same night or within a few days, so that material will still be familiar.

IX. How to Select a Textbook

Selecting a good textbook is an important skill, since a large portion of your medical education is acquired from books. If you choose the wrong book, you have dug yourself a deep hole. It will be difficult to read and less helpful for exams and clinical situations. On the other hand, a good text is more enjoyable to read and will serve you well as a source of information. In general, when selecting a book, it helps to "think like a child", eg. look for big print and lots of pictures.

Positive features

1. **Big print** - be nice to your eyes
2. **Pictures** - worth a thousand words
3. **Schematic diagrams** - more helpful than pictures
4. **Tables of data** - useful for DDx and quick review
5. **Concise** - "less is more", gives you the "big picture"
6. **Emphasis** - should be written for students at your level, check the preface
7. **Reputation** - ask older students, which books are best
8. **Format** - outline vs. prose, if prose should have short chapters and lots of subtitles
9. **Margins** - large enough to add your own notes

10. **Mnemonics** - facilitate learning and long term retention

11. **Practice Questions** - very helpful, eg. with the NMS books

12. **Size** - pocketsize clinical books function as a "peripheral brain" on the wards

X. Miscellaneous Tips

1. Be an active studier. Highlighting makes you become more involved in your studies because you must evaluate the material as you read it to decide which are the key words that should be highlighted. Using several different colors, the "rainbow method" of highlighting, helps you to categorize information and to separate important items that are located close to each other on the page. By underlining, paraphrasing and making margin notes you force yourself to further analyze and process the material.

2. Ask upperclass students for advice on how to approach difficult subjects/classes. Ask them to explain their opinions. You are searching for study hints that will work for you. The best advisors will be the ones that take their studies seriously, have similar study methods to your own and are able to explain why a particular method is useful for them.

CHAPTER 2
NATIONAL BOARDS

NATIONAL BOARDS/MEDICAL LICENSING EXAMINATIONS

I. INTRODUCTION

Currently the USMLE (United States Medical Licensing Examination) is being phased in to replace two existing examination sequences used in the medical licensing process: the Federation Licensing Examination (FLEX) and the certifying examinations of the National Board of Medical Examiners (NBME). Although the names have been changed the rules of the game are the same. Doing well on Part I /Step I is important for securing a good residency position, and passage of all three is required for medical licensure.

The NBME administers three national boards examinations, parts I, II, III. Currently the names of those examinations are being changed to USMLE steps I, II, III. Part I/Step I covers the basic sciences and is usually taken at the end of the 2nd year of medical school. Part II/Step II covers the core information of ob/gyn, pediatrics, psychiatry, medicine, surgery and public health, and is taken during the senior year. Part III/Step III is taken during the Spring of the internship year.

This discussion will focus on the NBME part I (NBpI)/USMLE Step I (MLEsI) examination because it is the most important and most difficult of the national boards exams. And NBpI/MLEsI scores are the primary screening device used by residency programs in competitive fields. This exam provides you with the opportunity and the motivation to review the basic sciences which form a foundation for the assimilation of clinical information during the 3rd year of medical school. It is useful to think of national boards part I as the final exam for the material covered in your basic science courses of anatomy, biochemistry, physiology, behavioral science, microbiology, pathology and pharmacology.

The best preparation is to study consistently and effectively all along during the first two years of medical school. Learn the material as well as you can during your regular medical school courses. However, a systematic determined effort during the last couple of months before the exam can make a big difference in terms of improved board scores. The general guidelines listed below will help you to prepare for the national boards part I examination.

II. Study Materials

Use your old notes!

It is best to use study materials (eg. books and notes) that are already familiar to you. This is a very important point. This enables you to review faster and remember better. For some topics it may be worthwhile to supplement with newly purchased or borrowed books. However, the best thing to do is to choose a good text and question book and to make good condensed notes during your regular medical school courses. That way most of your study time for NB/MLE will consist of reviewing familiar material, rather than trying to learn new information from new books. Make sure that you have a doable set of material, and then know it well. The concept of making good condensed notes is discussed in the section on study strategies.

III. Scheduling

Make a study schedule!

This will help you to pace yourself and to organize your study materials so that you can go through them in a systematic manner. Make sure to crank extra hard during the last 6 weeks because this will jack up your short term memory and improve your board scores. Some students find it helpful to list on a notecard the 7 major subjects in a vertical column and the subcategories in a horizontal row. For example, physiology subcategories include GI, CV, pulmonary and renal (see figure 1). Other methods found helpful for scheduling include using a large calendar to make a study schedule and/or making an outline of study topics.

Figure 1

1. Anatomy
    - Gross → upper extremity, lower extremity, back, thorax, etc.
    - Neuroanatomy, Histology, Embryology
2. Biochemistry
    - Carbohydrates, Lipids, Amino acids, Nucleic acids, etc.
3. Physiology
    - GI, CV, Pulmonary, Renal, Nerve-Muscle, etc.
4. Behavioral Science
    - Child development, Psychopathology, Medical sociology, etc.

5. Microbiology
   - Bacteria, Fungi, Viruses, Parasites, Immunology, etc.

6. Pathology
   - General, Respiratory, Renal, Endocrine, Hematopathology, etc.

7. Pharmacology
   - Autonomic nervous system, Cardiovascular, CNS, etc.

IV. SEQUENCE OF TOPICS

Although the specific sequence in which topics are studied is a matter of individual preference, the following suggestions have been found helpful by many students.

1. Begin by reviewing difficult, time consuming subjects from the M-I year such as cardiovascular physiology.

2. Topics that rely heavily on short-term memorization, such as most of biochemistry, are best covered in the last couple of weeks before the exam.

3. Some topics for a particular organ system, such as renal, seem to go well in sequence, eg. renal histology, renal physiology, renal pathology.

4. Topics that are relatively easy to study such as BS can be studied at night when your brain is too frazzled for other stuff.

5. Make sure to study topics that are especially clinically useful for the junior year of medical school, as well as for a career field in which you are interested. For example, you have to know the menstrual cycle backwards and forwards in detail for your ob/gyn clinical rotation. If you are interested in orthopedics you should give special attention for topics related to musculoskeletal metabolism and pathology, as well as the anatomy of UE, LE and back.

6. When the clock is running out and you only have study time for a few topics, choose topics that overlap between subject areas. For example, antibiotics are an important aspect of microbiology and pharmacology.

V. Question Books and Self Assessment

There are several ways to assess your progress. The only way to be sure that you really know something is to be able to discuss it without notes or to write a brief outline without notes or to do a question book. Immediately after studying a topic, do the associated questions (?'s). The first time around don't worry if the ?'s seem very difficult. They are designed to be that way. Even so, you should understand the key concept from the majority of ?'s. If not, then look it up. However, if you've already gone through the ?'s several times during your regular medical school courses, then you will quickly recognize the correct answers. Obviously, this is the best way to do it.

VI. ANATOMY

The anatomy section in NBpI consists of gross anatomy, neuroanatomy, histology and embryology. Gross and neuro are the most important. Most of your anatomy study time should be spent with these subjects. Histology and embryology are relatively minor subsections of the anatomy component.

GROSS ANATOMY

The choice of books for gross anatomy is a matter of individual preference. As with all other subjects the best study materials are those that you have already used in your regular medical school courses. Your class notes are a valuable source of information since they are closely connected with your classroom and laboratory experience. The main points from your class notes should be incorporated into your permanent set of condensed notes. Either the *NMS book of Anatomy* (ANMS) by Ernest April or the *Review of Gross Anatomy* by Ben Pansky can be used for making the framework of your permanent condensed notes. Although ANMS is better written and has excellent practice questions, Pansky is better for condensed notes because it has more illustrations, more margin space and an extremely user friendly format with pictures on the page opposite the corresponding text.

Mnemonics are another valuable study method for learning and remembering topics in gross anatomy. This book provides several gross anatomy mnemonics in the mnemonics section. It is useful to incorporate these mnemonics, as well as those you learn at your medical school into your condensed notes.

ANMS together with the Arco question book provide an excellent, comprehensive set of practice questions. In preparation for NBpI you should review your condensed notes, skim the Netter atlas and then do the above mentioned practice questions.

Listed bellow are mini-summaries of some of the most popular gross anatomy books.

1. *ANMS* by Ernest April
   - outline format
   - well written, but too long
   - good diagrams, but not enough in number
   - excellent study questions

2. *Review of Gross Anatomy* by Ben Pansky
   - extremely user friendly format with pictures on page opposite text
   - easy to skim through and to review from
   - lots of margin space for adding your own notes and drawings
   - pictures are mostly black and white drawings, many of which are well suited to being colored in by the student who so desires

3. *Atlas of Gross Anatomy* by Frank Netter
   - Frank Netter is the Michelangelo of medical illustration and this is his Sistine chapel. All medical students should own it.

4. Arco ? book: *Human Anatomy Review* by Montgomery and Singleton
   - excellent practice questions

5. *Anatomy Made Ridiculously Simple* by Stephen Goldberg
    - the best thing about this book is that it quickly gives you the big picture with clever drawings and imaginative, concise descriptions of some anatomical regions
    - Well written, but too simplified for your regular medical school course
    - However, many top students thought that it was enough for NBpI
    - it is best used as a supplement to some other text
    - in a pinch, it can be used as a quick review of gross anatomy

6. *Clinical Anatomy* by Richard Snell
    - Prose format
    - this book is way too long
    - excellent sections on clinical aspects of gross anatomy
    - Good practice questions which consist of word problems from clinical situations as well as typical basic science anatomy questions

NEUROANATOMY

Neuroanatomy Made Easy and Understandable (NMEU) by Michael Liebman is the best book for making condensed notes. *Neuroanatomy Made Ridiculously Simple* is an excellent supplemental text containing many clever drawings as well as a top notch set of practice problems. *The Medical Student's Guide to Top Board Scores* contains mnemonics for the spinal cord tracts and the cranial foramina that have been found helpful by many students. *The Ciba Atlas of Nervous System Anatomy and Physiology* is another masterpiece by Netter. For the neuroanatomy course at your medical school you should buy or borrow all three of these books. In preparation for NBpI you should review your condensed notes, skim through the pictures in the Netter Atlas and do the practice questions in NMEU and NMRS.

1. *Neuroanatomy Made Easy and Understandable* by Michael Liebman
    - This is a great book
    - well written and concise
    - excellent schematic diagrams which quickly give you the big picture
    - contains many short chapters which makes it easy to correlate with the classroom lectures at your school

2. *Neuroanatomy Made Ridiculously Simple* by Stephen Goldberg
    - well written, concise with clever diagrams
    - contains a top notch set of clinical practice problems
    - this is an excellent supplemental text

3. *Atlas of Nervous System Anatomy and Physiology* by Frank Netter
    - another masterpiece by Netter
    - just study the pictures, this book is great for looking up stuff from lecture material and laboratory assignments
    - I repeat, just study the pictures, do not waste time trying to read the text because it is out-of-date and the emphasis is not directed towards medical students

4. *Clinical Neuroanatomy* by Richard Snell
   - Prose format
   - this book is too long and too detailed-excellent sections on the clinical aspects of neuroanatomy which includes excellent practice problems
   - This is a good book if you want to use a long, comprehensive, prose text for neuroanatomy

HISTOLOGY

This is a relatively minor subsection of the anatomy component. Many students like to study the histology of an organ system just before going over its physiology. Histo serves as a good warm-up prior to cracking open the physiology set of study materials. These subjects go together well in sequence. If you don't have time to finish studying anatomy, it might be best to just skip over most of histology. However, make sure to cover the subtopics which overlap with other areas. Such as pathology of the skin. The *Textbook of Histology* by Wheater is highly regarded by many students.

1. *Functional Histology* by Wheater et al.
   - well written and concise
   - illustrations immediately adjacent to text
   - easy book to review from and go through quickly when preparing for exams

2. *Lange Series - Histology: Examination and Board Review* by Paulsen
   - excellent outline format
   - lots of practice questions

- however it has almost zero pictures and therefore should be used with an atlas such as *Functional Histology* by Wheater et al.

EMBRYOLOGY

This is a relatively minor subsection of the anatomy component. If you don't have time to finish studying anatomy, it might be best to just skim over most of embryology. However make sure to cover the subtopics which overlap with other areas such as gametogenesis and changes in the circulation at birth.

1. *Langman's Medical Embryology* by T.W. Sadler
   - excellent color illustrations
   - well written, concise chapter summaries

2. *Study Guide to Langman's Medical Embryology*
   - concise study guide to accompany text of same name
   - nice format

3. *Oklahoma Notes - Embryology* by Robert Coalson
   - concise chapters immediately followed by study questions

VII. BIOCHEMISTRY

It is best to study biochemistry during the last couple of weeks before NBpI because it relys heavily on short - term memorization. Mnemonics are extremely useful for biochemistry. Learn the biochemistry mnemonics in this book. Make up your own for additional topics. You should try to have mnemonics or at least highly condensed notes for all of the major biochemistry cycles and other topics.

It is worthwhile to study hard for biochemistry. The biochemistry questions on NBpI are the most straight forward of those for any subject, so that your study time pays off in terms of improved board scores. The three best books to study from are Stryer, Friedman and the McGraw Hill - Pretest Series question book. For your condensed notes you can use the Friedman text of biochemistry or else make your own separate collection of condensed notes on loose leaf paper which can be kept in a folder or a ringbinder notebook. As you study the different subtopics of biochemistry during your preparation for NBpI, you should be further editing the condensed notes made during your regular medical school course and/or making new summary notes. Then during the last week before NBpI skim over these summary notes. This will keep the material fresh in your mind.

1. *Biochemistry* by Lupert Stryer
   - beautifully written, however quite long
   - you need to use it during your regular medical school course, in order to make it useful in preparing for NBpI
   - excellent color diagrams
   - excellent sections on molecular biology

2. *Biochemistry* by Friedman
   - an excellent review of biochemistry for NBpI
   - well written concise chapters
   - excellent study questions
   - the DNA/RNA/protein synthesis section is deficient (you can supplement with Stryer)

3. McGraw Hill - Pretest Series - *Biochemistry*
    - excellent study questions

PHYSIOLOGY

Physiology is a difficult, time consuming subject. It is considered by many students to be the most difficult subject of the basic sciences because it is the most conceptual. To do well in physiology you have to understand the concept for each organ system and be able to solve test problems that require a very careful, step-by-step, well reasoned analytical approach. Rote memorization alone will not suffice. Also some physiology problems require mathematical calculations, and medical students, of course, hate math. That is why we went to medical school instead of into some other area of science.

In addition to being conceptual, physiology is also time consuming. You have to get after it early. Many students, including myself found it best to start out with physiology topics, such as CV physio, pulmonary physio and GI physio, for the study surge that begins during the last few months before NBpI. You want to get some of this difficult stuff out of the way. Starting early helps you to be calm (less stressed) because you start studying while the test is still a ways away. Then when it gets closer you know that you've already done some studying.

Although time consuming your hard work in physiology is a highly rewarding investment for the future. Physiology provides you with a foundation that helps to prepare you for pharmacology, pathology and clinical medicine. In fact, during your M-2 year it is worthwhile to try to review the physiology of an organ system just prior to studying its pathology, especially with subjects where there is a lot of overlap such as CV physio and CV path.

The Little Brown Series Book of Physiology by Hsu et al. is the most highly recommended text. However, *Review of Medical Physiology* by Ganong has also been popular with many students. The McGraw-Hill Pretest series question book is excellent. The Arco question book has good practice questions, but it is quite long and is considered too detailed by some students.

1. Little Brown Series Book of Physiology by Hsu et al.
    - this is the most highly recommended text
    - concise
    - contains some practice questions

2. *Review of Medical Physiology* by Ganong
    - popular with many students

3. McGraw-Hill Pretest Series Question book by Dise
    - excellent questions

4. *Human Physiology Examination Review* (The Arco question book) by Shephard
    - good questions
    - excellent format with answers immediately following the question
    - lots of short chapters which facilitates correlation between study notes and practice problems
    - quite long and considered too detailed by some students

5. *Textbook of Medical Physiology* by Guyton
    - popular among many students who felt that it explained things well
    - well written and enjoyable to read, but it is too long
    - prose format is difficult to review from

- some students have found it particularly helpful to put lots of study notes in the margins

6. National Medical Series (NMS)Book of Physiology by Bullock et al.
   - outline format
   - contains practice questions

7. *Color Atlas of Physiology* by Agememnon Despopoulos and Stefan Silbernagel
   - nice diagrams which provide the big picture
   - however it has suffered a lot in the translation from a foreign language which makes the printed text virtually worthless
   - nice portable, pocket size which makes this the kind of book you can skim through while taking the train to school or riding an exercycle

BEHAVIORAL SCIENCE

Behavioral science is a relatively easy subject. Many of the behavioral science questions on NBpI can be divined by common sense. Watch *The Simpsons* to get these. However to be on the safe side a textbook is recommended. The most popular book is *BS for the Boreds*. It is a very concise book which provides a good framework for making one's condensed notes by supplementing with material from your classroom lecture course. It is recommended that you put lots of notes in the margins and that you look up stuff which seems important even if it is only briefly mentioned in *BS for the Boreds*.

1. *Behavioral Science for the Boreds* by Frederick Sierles
   - very concise
   - a good framework for making condensed notes

2. NMS Book - *Behavioral Science* by Wiener
   - outline format
   - contains study questions
   - this book is popular with some students who did very well in behavioral science

MICROBIOLOGY

If you have made good condensed notes for microbiology, eg. by putting classroom lecture summary notes into the margins of Microbiology Synopsis, it should be relatively easy to review for NBpI. Other variables in your favor include the fact that microbiology relies heavily on memorization/word association, and it is usually taught during the M-2 year. The key strategies for doing well in microbiology are understanding the classification system and memorizing the distinguishing features for individual microorganisms. Classification is the framework around which Microbiology Synopsis is designed and for each individual bug there is usually only 1-to-5 things to know about it.

The Microbiology Synopsis within this text quickly gives you the big picture and provides you with a concise overview of clinical microbiology. The Lange series book-*Microbiology and Immunology Examination and Board Review* by Levinson and Jawetz is extremely popular as a concise reference text, and it also contains lots of study questions. The *Microbiology and Immunology* text from Oklahoma notes series is also quite popular. It is very concise, has a user friendly format and contains practice questions. However the best study questions are to be found in the Medical Examination Review series and Arco series questions books for microbiology.

1. *Microbiology Synopsis* by P. Thomas Rogers
    - ultraconcise, a good framework for condensed notes
    - located within this text
    - quickly provides you with the big picture

2. Lange series - *Microbiology and Immunology Examination and Board Review* by Levinson and Jawetz
    - extremely popular reference text
    - contains practice questions

3. *Oklahoma Notes - Microbiology* by Hyde
    - well liked for its user friendly format
    - concise

4. *Medical Examination Review - Microbiology Question Book* by Kim
    - concise
    - excellent practice questions

5. Arco? Book - *Microbiology and Immunology Review* by Rothfield
    - more extensive, relatively comprehensive
    - excellent practice questions

PATHOLOGY

Pathology is considered by many students to be the most interesting of the second year subjects. It is fascinating to learn about basic disease processes and how specific organ systems are affected. However, it is definitely the most difficult and most time consuming of the M-2 year subjects. Although memorization is important, it also relies heavily on concepts and on accumulated knowledge from previous courses such as physiology and histology.

Due to the content of the subject matter and the volume of the material, organization is the key to doing well in pathology.

Follow the outlines from the *Pocket Book of Pathology* by Robbins et al. and use these outlines to make concise summary notes. Some students may prefer to use the NMS book of Pathology by LiVoisi et al. as their primary study source and framework for condensed notes. These condensed notes are great for quick review. In addition these outline formatted summary notes facilitate memory by helping you to think clearly and systematically about the mechanisms and manifestations of disease.

Although you might wish to impress members of the opposite sex, it is strongly recommended that you do not use one of the big, hardcover type pathology textbooks as your primary study source. If you want to buy a hardcover text to use as a reference, get the intermediate sized *Basic Pathology* (Baby Robbins) by Robbins and Kumar. However, the larger books are notoriously long winded and ill suited to the needs of second year students. You will be much happier and will get much better grades by using a concise, streamlined text that gets good mileage per paragraph and is oriented towards second year students.

Another important suggestion is to do lots and lots of study questions. You should do the practice questions in *Pathologic Basis of Disease, Self-Assessment and Review* by Compton which serves as the study guide to the textbook *Pathologic Basis of Disease* by Robbins et al. For those of you with the time and the inclination, the practice questions in the Arco question book are also excellent.

1. *The Pocket Companion to Robbins Pathologic Basis of Disease* by Robbins, Cotran and Kumar
    - concise
    - excellent outlines at the beginning of each chapter
    - very popular among students

2. *National Medical Series - Pathology* by LiVoisi
    - outline format
    - contains practice questions

3. *Basic Pathology* by Robbins and Kumar
    - Intermediate sized pathology textbook
    - somewhat verbose, but useful as a reference text

4. *Pathology* by Rubin and Farber
    - awesome illustrations
    - excellent diagrams
    - However, the text in the first edition is long winded and poorly written. This might improve with subsequent editions.

5. *Pathologic Basis of Disease, Self-Assessment and Review* by Compton
    - excellent practice questions

6. Arco ? books
    → *General Pathology Review* by Lewis and Kerwin
    → *Systemic Pathology Review* by Lewis and Kerwin
    - excellent practice questions

PHARMACOLOGY

Pharmacology is another subject which relies heavily on memorization. The most popular study approaches are flash cards, freehand outlines and condensed notes within a book. Students have been able to do very well with any of these methods.

PDQ Pharmacology by Johnson has an outline format and provides an excellent framework for making condensed notes. This gives you a permanent set of well organized summary notes which facilitates quick referencing and review. Flashcards are also great for quick review, but are often awkward for use as a reference.

It is also important to do lots of study questions. The Lange series - *Pharmacology: Examination and Board Review* by Katzung and Trevor is an excellent book with lots of short chapters that are immediately followed by practice questions. Note this is the short course review book with lots of practice questions which is something completely different than the large reference text that is also written by Katzung. Some students found the NMS book of Pharmacology useful as a reference text. The most highly recommended question book is the Arco series question book.

1. *PDQ Pharmacology* by Johnson
    - ultra-concise with an outline format
    - excellent framework for making condensed notes

2. Lange series - *Pharmacology: Examination and Board Review* by Katzung and Trevor
    - an excellent book
    - lots of concise, short chapters followed immediately by study questions

3. NMS book *Pharmacology* by Leonard Jacob
   - useful as a reference text
   - contains practice questions

4. Arco series question book by Ellis
   - excellent questions
   - lots of short chapters which makes it easier to do practice sections right after you have studied a topic

Chapter 3
M-1 Mnemonics

ANATOMY MNEMONICS

NERVE INJURIES IN THE UPPER EXTREMITY *ANK

Lesions of the radial nerve, ulnar nerve or median nerve have a characteristic effect on the hand which can be remembered by the mnemonic, "**DR. CUMA**".

D • Drop wrist

R • Radial n

C • Clawhand

U • Ulnar n

M • Median n

A • Ape hand

BONES OF THE WRIST *ANK

The mnemonic for the bones of the wrist is "**Some Lovers Try Positions That They Can't Handle**".

Some	→	Scaphoid
Lovers	→	Lunate
Try	→	Triquetrum
Positions	→	Pisiform
That	→	Trapezium
They	→	Trapezoid
Can't	→	Capitate
Handle	→	Hamate

AXILLARY ARTERY *ANK

The mnemonic for the branches of the axillary artery is "**Sally Thompson Loves Sex and Pot**".

Sally	→	Superior thoracic
Thompson	→	Thoracoacromial
Loves	→	Lateral thoracic
Sex	→	Subscapular
And	→	Anterior humeral circumflex
Pot	→	Posterior humeral circumflex

ROTATOR CUFF MUSCLES *ANK

The rotator cuff muscles help to stabilize the shoulder joint. The mnemonic for the rotator cuff muscle is "**SITS**". For example, when an athlete, such as former Chicago Bears quarterback Jim McMahon, has a rotator cuff injury he sits out the game.

S • Supraspinatus

I • Infraspinatus

T • Teres Minor

S • Subscapularis

EXTERNAL CAROTID ARTERY

The mnemonic for the branches of the external carotid artery is "**SAL-FO-PSM**". The long form of this is **S**ome **A**dolescents **L**ove **F**ellatio, **O**thers **P**refer **S** and **M**.

- **S** • Superior thyroid
- **A** • Ascending pharyngeal
- **L** • Lingual
- **F** • Facial
- **O** • Occipital
- **P** • Posterior auricular
- **S** • Superficial temporal
- **M** • Maxillary

THE TRIANGULAR SPACE *ANK

The triangular space in the shoulder region is bounded by the "**3-T's**".

T • Triceps

T • Teres minor

T • Teres major

MITOSIS *ANK

The stages of mitosis can be remembered by the mnemonic, "**IP-MAT**"

I • Interphase

P • Prophase

M • Metaphase

A • Anaphase

T • Telophase

CHROMOSOME NOMENCLATURE

The mnemonic for chromosome nomenclature is "**NARBS**", which stands for chromosome Number, Arm, **R**egion, **B**and and **S**ubband. For example 1p23.4 represents the 1st chromosome, short arm/p arm ("p" for petite), 2nd region, 3rd band, 4th subband.

N • Number of chromosome

A • Arm

R • Region

B • Band

S • Subband

THE BRACHIAL PLEXUS

You will most often encounter pt's w/brachial plexus injuries in the newborn nursery, emergency room and orthopedic clinic. The brachial plexus is comprised of **R**oots, **T**runks and **C**ords which can be remembered by the mnemonic "**RTC**". The roots are the anterior rami of spinal nerves C5 to T1. The roots join together to form trunks, and the trunks give rise to the cords. The cords are named for their position relative to the axillary artery. The cords give rise to the terminal branches which can be remembered by the mnemonic, "**MARMU**".

R • Roots → C5 to T1
- → 1. Dorsal scapular
- 2. Long thoracic

T • Trunks → Upper
- → 1. Suprascapular
- 2. n to Subclavius

Middle
Lower

C • Cords → Lat
- → 1. Lateral Pectoral

→ Post
- → 1. Upper & Lower Subscapular
- 2. Thoracordorsal

→ Med
- → 1. Medial Pectoral
- 2. Medial Brachial & antebrachial cutaneous

THE BRACHIAL PLEXUS

Terminal Branches

M • Median

A • Axillary

R • Radial

M • Musculocutaneous

U • Ulnar

HEPATIC PORTAL CIRCULATION

The major vessels of the portal circulation are shaped like a "chair". With this framework in mind, one can more easily visualize the location of other portal vein tributaries and anatomical structures. The portal circulation has important anastomoses with the esophageal veins, the paraumbilical veins, the middle rectal and inferior rectal veins as well as the retroperitonal tributaries of the inferior vena cava.

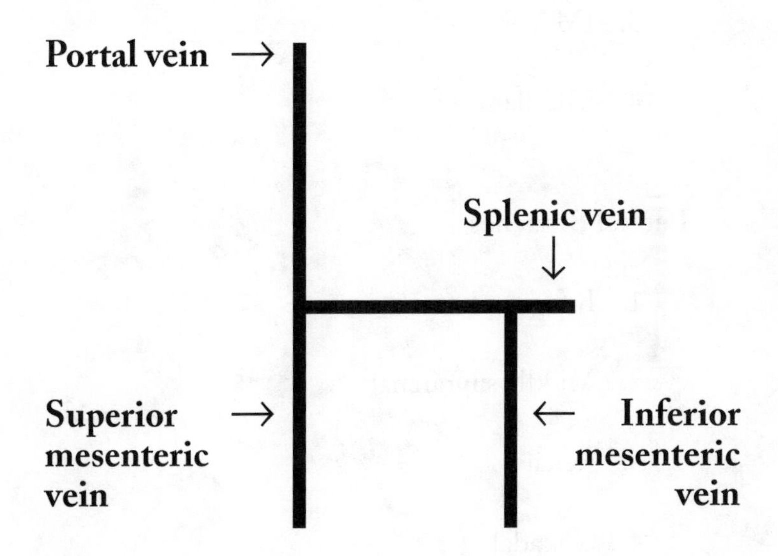

ABDOMINAL AORTA *ANK

The branches of the abdominal aorta can be remembered by the rule of 4's.

Midline Branches

1. Celiac trunk
2. SMA
3. IMA
4. Middle sacral

Lateral Branches

1. Inferior phrenic
2. Middle suprarenal
3. Renal
4. Gonadal

Posterior

1. Lumbar → 4 paired arteries

SUPERIOR MESENTERIC ARTERY

The branches of the superior mesenteric artery can be remembered by the mnemonic, "**I3RMA**".

I • Inferior pancreaticoduodenal artery

• Intestinal arteries (jejunal & ileal)

• Ileocolic artery

R • Right colic

M • Middle colic

A • Anastomoses via marginal artery

NECK TRIANGLES

The Triangles of the neck can be remembered by the mnemonic, **M3-C-O2**.

Anterior Triangle

M • Mental (submental)

M • Mandibular (submandibular)

M • Muscular

C • Carotid

O • Occipital

O • Omoclavicular

CAROTID SHEATH

The contents of the carotid sheath can be remembered by the mnemonic, "**VNA**".

V • Vein → internal jugular

N • Nerve → vagus

A • Artery → carotid

CRANIAL SUTURES

The mnemonic for the cranial sutures is "**CBS** λ", which stands for **C**oronal suture, **B**regma, **S**agittal suture, **L**ambdoid suture and **L**ambda.

C • Coronal suture

B • Bregma

S • Sagittal suture

λ • Lambdoid suture

• Lambda

SPINAL CORD TRACTS

The mnemonic for the most important spinal cord tracts is "**P-SLAC**". This represents the **P**osterior columns (= fasiculus gracilis and cuneatus), **S**pinocerebeller tract, **L**ateral spinothalamic tract (LSTT), **A**nterior spinothalamic tract (ASTT) and the **C**orticospinal tract.

	Tract	Function	Site of Crossover
P •	Posterior columns	fine touch conscious proprioception vibratory sense	medulla
S •	Spinocerebellar tract	muscle tone and unconscious proprioception	ipsilateral
L •	LSTT	pain and temperature	spinal cord
A •	ASTT	crude touch	spinal cord
C •	Corticospinal tract	voluntary motor	medulla

Cranial Foramina

The mnemonic for the cranial foramina is "**ESTO**", which stands for the following bones, **E**thmoid, **S**phenoid, **T**emporal and **O**ccipital.

Bone		Foramen/site of passage	Cranial nerve or other structure
E •	Ethmoid	cribiform plate	1
S •	Sphenoid	optic canal	2
		superior orbital fissure	3, 4, 6 & V1
		foramen rotundum	V2
		foramen ovale	V3
		foramen spinosum	middle meningeal artery
T •	Temporal	internal auditory meatus	7 & 8
O •	Occipital	jugular foramen	9, 10, 11 & internal jugular vein,
		foramen magnum	brainstem, vertebral arteries
		hypoglossal canal	12

LIGAMENTS OF THE VERTEBRAL COLUMN

The mnemonic for the ligaments of the vertebral column is "**SIF - PA**".

S • Supraspinal

I • Infraspinal

F • Flavum

P • Posterior longitudinal

A • Anterior longitudinal

THE DISTAL SPINAL CORD

The magic number is "**142**" for the anatomy of the distal spinal cord.

1 → The spinal cord ends at $\underline{L_1}$

4 → The $\underline{L_4}$ interspace is a good site for doing a lumbar puncture.

2 → $\underline{S_2}$ is where the subarachnoid space terminates.

BONES OF THE ORBIT

The mnemonic for the bones of the orbit is "**FELM PO3SZ**", which is pronounced similiar to the phrase "film pose". Note: the "O3" stands for optic canal and orbital fissures (superior and inferior).

F • Frontal

E • Ethmoid

L • Lacrimal

M • Maxillary

P • Palatine

O • Optic canal and Orbital fissures

S • Sphenoid

Z • Zygomatic

ANATOMY OF THE EYEBALL

The magic number is "**3**" when studying the anatomy of the eyeball because the eyeball has three coats, three chambers and three main structures for refraction and vision.

I. **Three Coats**

1. Outer fibrous coat = Sclera and cornea
2. Middle Vascular coat = Uvea = Choroid, ciliary body and iris
3. Inner retinal coat = Retina

II. **Three Chambers**

1. Anterior chamber
2. Posterior chamber
3. Vitreous chamber

III. **Three Main Structures for Refraction and Vision**

1. Cornea → crude focus
2. Lens → fine focus
3. Retina → contains photoreceptors

THE MUSCLES OF THE EYE

The magic number is "**3**" when studying the muscles of the eye because there are three muscles for the eyelid, three intraocular muscles (IOM) for the eyeball, and three nerves innervate the extraocular muscles (EOM) of the eyeball.

LR6(SO4)3

I. **Muscles of the Eyelid**

1. Levator palpebrae superioris
2. Superior tarsal (= Muller's muscle)
3. Orbicularis oculi (palpebrae portion)

II. **IOM**

1. Ciliary (lens)
2. Constrictor pupillae
3. Dilator pupillae

III. **EOM**

1. CN#6 → Lateral rectus → LR_6
2. CN#4 → Superior oblique → SO_4
3. CN#3 → the other EOM

PARANASAL SINUSES

The mnemonic for the paranasal sinuses is "**FEMS**".

- **F** • Frontal
- **E** • Ethmoid
- **M** • Maxillary
- **S** • Sphenoid

BIOCHEMISTRY MNEMONICS

GLYCOLYSIS (I)

Glycolysis is the most important pathway for glucose (glc) metabolism. It is the sequence of reactions that produces 2 ATP's, 2 NADH's and converts glc into pyruvate (pyr). You should memorize it paying special attention to the sequence of glycolytic intermediates and enzymes, the reactions that produce ATP or NADH and the regulatory/control reactions (rxn's).

The sequence of rxn's can be remembered by the mnemonic, **(661) 63*-1332**. This is the "phone number of Mr. Glycolysis". The * represents DHAP in which the Ⓟ is not numbered. Each number represents the location of the Ⓟ on the glycolytic intermediates. This will enable you to list these compounds in order.

Most of the enzymes are named after their associated substrate or product and according to the type of rxn they catalyze. Thus, once you write out the sequence of glycolytic intermediates, it is relatively easy to recall the names of the enzymes. Hexokinase, PFK and Pyr Kinase are the main regulatory enzymes. They catalyze irreversible rxn's. The 1st diagram is a list of the glycolytic intermediates. The 2nd diagram includes the enzymes and the locations of where ATP and NADH are produced or utilized.

GLYCOLYSIS (II)

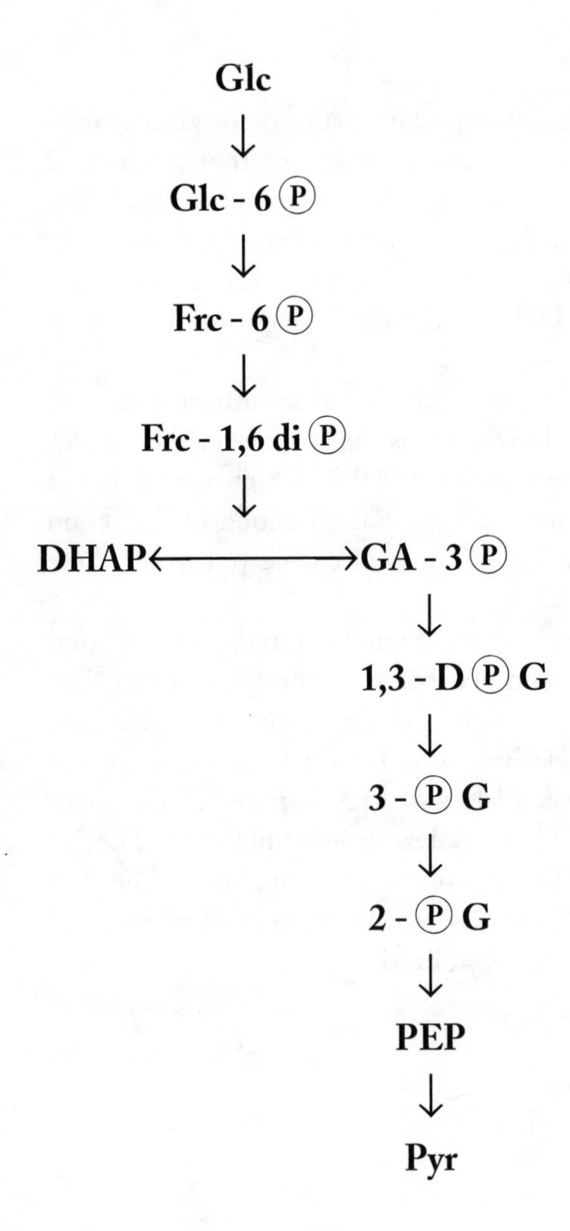

GLYCOLYSIS (III)

Glc

↓ (Hexokinase) lose ATP

Glc - 6 Ⓟ

↓ (Isomerase)

Frc - 6 Ⓟ

↓ (PFK) lose ATP

Frc - 1,6 di Ⓟ

↓ (Aldolase)

DHAP ⟷ GA - 3 Ⓟ

(Triose Isomerase)

↓ (GA - dehydrog) gain NADH

1,3 - D Ⓟ G

↓ (PG Kinase) gain ATP

3 - Ⓟ G

↓ (Mutase)

2 - Ⓟ G

↓ (Enolase)

PEP

↓ (Pyr Kinase) gain ATP

Pyr

TRICARBOXYLIC ACID CYCLE (I)

The TCA cycle is the final common pathway for the oxidative metabolism of carbohydrates, amino acids and lipids. It is the sequence of rxn's that for each turn yields 3 NADH, one FADH, one GTP and two CO_2. The intermediates can be remembered by the mnemonic, **CIA5-S+S-FMO**.

Each letter represents a TCA cycle intermediate. The + sign represents the production of GTP and the fact that Succinyl CoA comes before Succinate. In terms of memorizing the cycle Alpha-KG is the most important compound. It is the only compound with five carbons and CO_2 is given off immediately prior to and following the presence of alpha-KG. Each turn of the cycle begins with a two carbon structure (acetyl CoA) and later loses two carbons in the form of CO_2. The first diagram emphasizes that alpha-KG is the only compound with five carbons. The second diagram is a list of the TCA cycle intermediates and shows where NADH, CO_2, GTP and FADH are produced.

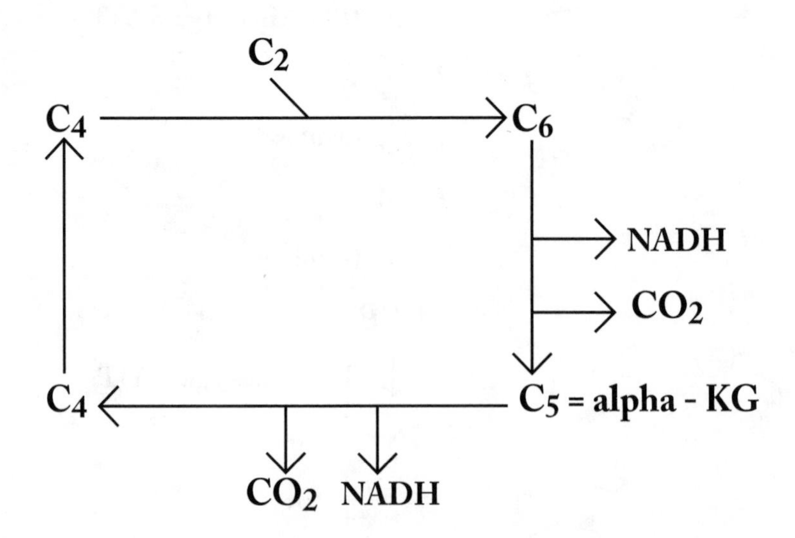

TRICARBOXYLIC ACID CYCLE (II)

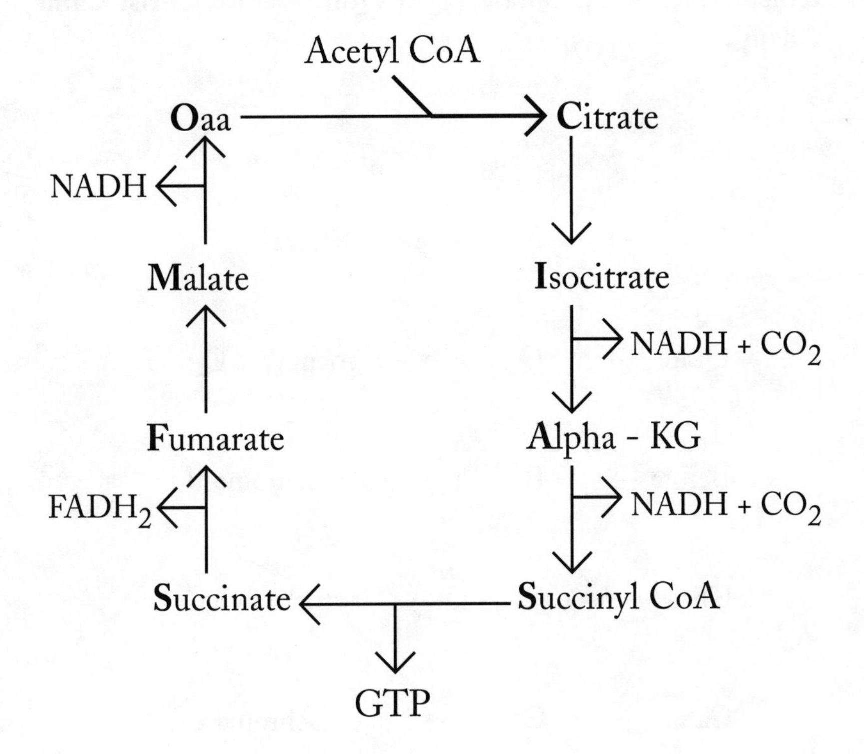

CIA
S + S
FMO

THE ELECTRON TRANSPORT CHAIN

The components of the electron transport chain can be remembered by the phrase, "**Not Quite Before Christ Came Adam**".

Not	→	**N**	→	NADH
Quite	→	**Q**	→	coenzyme Q
Before	→	**B**	→	cytochrome B
Christ	→	**C**	→	cytochrome C_1
Came	→	**C**	→	cytochrome C
Adam	→	**A**	→	cytochrome A

ESSENTIAL AMINO ACIDS *ANK

The essential amino acids can be remembered by the mnemonic, "**SABBT**". The amino acids that are underlined are nonessential but are synthesized from essential amino acids.

S •	Sulfur	→	Met, Cys
A •	Aromatic	→	Phe, Tyr, Trp
B •	Basic	→	Arg, Lys, His
B •	Branched	→	Val, Ile, Leu
T •	Threonine		

THE UREA CYCLE

† R. WILLIAM BETCHER M.D.

The urea cycle can be remembered by the mnemonic, **"Ordinarily Careless Crappers Are Also Frivolous About Urination"**.

Ordinarily	→	Ornithine
Careless	→	Carbamoyl Ⓟ
Crappers	→	Citrulline
Are	→	Aspartate
Also	→	Argininosuccinate
Frivolous	→	Fumarate
About	→	Arginine
Urination	→	Urea

† A Student to Student Guide to Medical School, (Boston: Little Brown Co., 1985)

CHOLESTEROL SYNTHESIS *ANK

The mnemonic for Cholesterol synthesis is "**Ah! Ah! Help Me! - Plan In Diet Good Food - Stay Low (in) Cholesterol**".

Ah!	→	Acetyl CoA
Ah!	→	Acetoacetyl CoA
Help	→	HMG CoA
Me!	→	Mevalonate
Plan	→	Ⓟ mevalonate
In	→	Isopentenyl pyro Ⓟ
Diet	→	Dimethylallyl pyro Ⓟ
Good	→	Geraynl pyro Ⓟ
Food	→	Farnesyl pyro Ⓟ
Stay	→	Squalene
Low (in)	→	Lanosterol
Cholesterol	→	Cholesterol

LIPIDOSES

The mnemonic for Lipidoses/disorders of sphingomyelin metabolism is "**SHAG3**".

	Enzyme deficiency	Disease
S	• Sphingomyelinase	Niemann-Pick disease
H	• Hexoseaminidase	Tay-Sachs disease
A	• Aryl Sulfatase	Metachromatic leukodystrophy
G	• Galactosidase (α)	Fabry's disease
	• Galactosidase (β)	Krabbes disease (=Globoid cell leukodystrophy)
	• Glucocerebrosidase	Gaucher's disease

FAT SOLUBLE VITAMINS *ANK

The fat soluble vitamins are easily remembered by the mnemonic, "**ADEK**".

A • A → deficiency can cause night blindness, xeropthalmia, blindness and follicular hyperkeratosis

D • D → deficiency in children causes rickets deficiency in adults causes osteomalacia

E • E → deficiency has been associated w/hemolytic anemia in premature infants

K • K → deficiency can cause hemorrhage

PELLAGRA *ANK

Pellagra is caused by a clinically significant deficiency of niacin or its precursor tryptophan. Pellagra is characterstically seen in persons whose diet consists mainly of corn, because corn is low in niacin and tryptophan. It is also occasionally seen in malnourished chronic alcoholics. The clinical features of pellagra can be remembered by "**5-D's**".

D • Deficiency of niacin

D • Diarrhea

D • Dermatitis

D • Dementia

D • Damage/inflammation of tongue which becomes bright red, swollen and painful

VITAMIN B_{12} & FOLATE

A deficiency of vitamin B_{12} or of folate can cause megaloblastic anemia. In addition, deficiency of vitamin B_{12} can also cause severe neurological damage in the spinal cord which is called subacute combined degeneration. Green leafy vegetables (foliage) are a good source of folate. Animal products such as beef are a good source of vitamin B_{12}.

"B"$_{12}$ → from **"B"**eef

"F"olate → from **"F"**oliage

PHYSIOLOGY MNEMONICS

LUNG VOLUMES

The lung volumes can be remembered by the mnemonic, "**LITERS**". TLC is six liters, which is equal to the sum of IRV, TV, ERV, and RV. The numbers listed below are useful approximations. Lung volumes will vary depending on the pt's size, build and pulmonary condition.

L • Lung Volumes

I • IRV = 3,000 ml

T • TV = 500 ml

E • ERV = 1,250 ml

R • RV = 1,250 ml

S • Six liters = 6,000 ml

SIDE EFFECTS OF CORTICOSTEROIDS

* DR. JOHN STOGIN M.D.

The side effects of corticosteroids can be remembered by the mnemonic, "**MOM'S PIG SACK**".

M • Myopathy

O • Osteoporosis

M •
Masked Symptomatology
S •

P • Personality changes

I • Infection

G • Growth retardation

S • Skin changes

A • Abnormal glucose tolerance

C • Cushingoid features

K • K^+ deficit

THE LIMBIC SYSTEM

The functions of the Limbic system can be remembered by the "**5-F's**".

F • Feeding

F • Fighting

F • Fear

F • Sex

F • not Forgetting (eg. the hippocampus appears to be involved with recent memory)

THE CEREBELLUM

In order to become a MVP caliber athlete one must have a cerebellum that functions well. The mnemonic for the functions of the cerebellum is "**MVP**".

M • Motor fine control (coordination)

V • Vestibular function (equilibrium)

P • Posture and muscle tone

BEHAVIORAL SCIENCE MNEMONICS

MENTAL STATUS EXAM (I)

The mental status exam (MSE) is to psychiatry what the physical exam is to internal medicine.The evaluation of any patient with a psychiatric disorder should always include the MSE.

When someone is an expert at something they are sometimes referred to as "Joe-expert" in that field. Using the same concept, an expert with the MSE may be referred to as "Joe-Mental-Status Exam." An abbreviation of this term is used to represent the components of the MSE. Thus the mnemonic for the MSE is **"JO-M-STA4T"**.

This mnemonic will make it easier to conduct the MSE efficiently and effectively. The four terms starting with the letter "A", Appearance, Attitude, Activity, Affect and mood should be listed at the beginning of your MSE write up. Notice that some of the components have been further subcategorized. However, you will learn much more about all of these during your physical diagnosis course and your psychiatry clerkship.

MENTAL STATUS EXAM (II)

J • Judgement

O • Orientation

M • Memory

→ 1. IR = immediate recall
2. ST = short term
3. LT = long term

S • Speech

→ **R** = Rate
A = Amount
T = Tone
E = Echolalia, dysarthria, and any other abnormalities

T • Thought process

→ **F** • Flight of ideas
L • Loose associations
T • Tangentiality, circumstantiality perseveration, blocking

A4 • Appearance, Attitude, Activity, Affect and mood

T • Thought content

→ **S** • Suicidal
H • Homicidal
O • Obsessions
D • Delusions

FREUD'S DEVELOPMENTAL STAGES

The psychosexual development stages of Freud can be remembered by the mnemonic, "**FOAPE-LaG**" (pronounced FOAPY-LaG). The approximate ages at which these stages occur is also listed.

F • Freud's developmental stages

O • Oral → Infancy (0 - 1.5 yrs)

A • Anal → Toddlerhood (1.5 - 3 yrs)

P • Phallic → Preschool (3 - 6 yrs)

E • oEdipal/Electra → Preschool

L • Latency → Elementary School (6 - 12 yrs)

(a)

G • Genital → Adolescence & Adulthood

ERICKSON'S DEVELOPMENTAL STAGES

Erickson's developmental task stages can be remembered by the mnemonic, "**TAFI-PI**". The letter "F" represents the number 'four' because there are four task stages that start with the letter "I".

T • Trust v.s. mistrust → Infancy

A • Autonomy v.s. shame & doubt → Toddlerhood

F • Four I's

I • 1. Initiative v.s. guilt → Preschool

2. Industry v.s. inferiority → Elememtary school

3. Identity v.s. role diffusion → Adolescence

4. Intimacy v.s. isolation → Young adulthood

P • Productivity v.s. stagnation (generativity) → Later adulthood

I • Integrity v.s. despair → Old age

WERNICKE-KORSAKOFF SYNDROME

The Wernicke-Korsakoff syndrome is an alcohol associated neurologic disorder caused by a deficiency of thiamine. Wernicke's encephalopathy is the acute phase and its clinical features can be remembered by the mnemonic, "**COAT**". Korsakoff's psychosis is the chronic phase and its characteristic findings are represented by the mnemonic, "**RACK**".

C • Confusion

O • Opthalmoplegia

A • Ataxia

T • Thiamine is an important aspect of Tx

R • Retrograde amnesia
(↓ recall of some old memories)

A • Anterograde amnesia
(↓ ability to form new memories)

C • Confabulation

K • Korsakoff's psychosis

THE STAGES OF DYING * DR. KUBLER-ROSS

The stages of dying as defined by Dr. Kubler-Ross can be remembered by the mnemonic, "**DAB-DA**".

D • Denial

A • Anger

B • Bargaining

D • Depression

A • Acceptance

ANOREXIA NERVOSA

The mnemonic for the clinical features of anorexia nervosa is "**ANOR EXIC**".

A • Adolescent females

• Amenhorrea

N • NGT alimentation is reserved for the most severe cases

O • Obsession with losing weight

• fear of becoming fat although underweight

• distorted body image → feels fat even though emaciated

R • Refusal to eat ≥ 5% die

E • Electrolyte abnormalities eg. ↓ K^+, cardiac arrh

X • ↑ eXercise

I • Intelligence often above average

• Induced vomiting

C • Cathartic & diuretic abuse may occur

• Carotenemia

NARCOLEPSY

Narcolepsy is one of the hypersomnia disorders. Its clinical features can be remembered by the mnemonic, "**CRASH**".

C • Cataplexy

R • REM onset sleep

A • Adolescent onset (usually)

S • Sleep attacks,
Sleep paralysis,
excessive daytime sleepiness

H • Hypnagogic hallucinations

SENSITIVITY & SPECIFICITY

The definitions of sensitivity and specificity are notoriously difficult to remember. The following examples of ways to write out these equations have proven helpful for many students.

$$\text{Sensitivity} = \frac{\text{True} \oplus}{\text{Truly} \oplus} = \frac{\text{T}\oplus}{\text{T}\oplus + \text{F}\ominus}$$

$$\text{Specificity} = \frac{\text{True} \ominus}{\text{Truly} \ominus} = \frac{\text{T}\ominus}{\text{T}\ominus + \text{F}\oplus}$$

ALCOHOL WITHDRAWL

Alcohol withdrawal is potentially lethal. The clinical features of alcohol withdrawal can be remembered by the mnemonic, "**SHIT**".

S • Shakes, Sweats, Seizures, Stomach pains (eg. nausea & vomiting)

H • Hallucinosis (eg. auditory)

I • Increased vitals signs & Insomnia

T • Tremens → delirium tremens (potentially lethal)

Chapter 4
M-2 Mnemonics

PHARMACOLOGY MNEMONICS

NARCOTIC ANALGESICS

Narcotic analgesics such as morphine, meperidine, codeine and propoxyphene have many important clinical uses. However, one must be careful to make sure that pt's do not get sucked in by the "VAACUUM" of narcotic side effects and addictive properties.

V • Vomiting

A • Analgesia

A • Antitussive

C • Constipation

U • Under = sedation

U • Under = respiratory depression

M • Miosis

BENZODIAZEPINES

† R. WILLIAM BETCHER M.D.

The main pharmacologic actions of benzodiazepines can be remembered by the mnemonic, "SCAM".

S • Sedation

C • anti - Convulsant

A • anti - Anxiety

M • Muscle relaxation

† A Student to Student Guide to Medical School, (Boston: Little Brown Co., 1985)

PATHOLOGY MNEMONICS

MALIGNANT BREAST TUMORS

There is a high incidence of breast carcinoma among women in the United States. Risk factors include positive family Hx, menstrual Hx characterised by ↑ unopposed estrogen (↑UOE), as well as fibrocystic change with atypical hyperplasia. Breast carcinoma may present as a firm mass, retraction of the nipple, fixation of breast tissue to the chest wall, dimpling of the skin or skin edema.

The mnemonic for the DDx of malignant breast tumors is "**DIMPLE**". Infiltrating ductal CA (eg. scirrhous) is the most common. Inflammatory CA implies invasion of the dermal lymphatics and has a poor prognosis. Medullary CA is a/w a lymphocytic infiltrate and has an above average prognosis. Mucinous (colloid) CA is a mucin producing tumor that also has an above average prognosis. Cytosarcoma phyllodes is a giant fibroadenoma that is usually benign but may undergo malignant transformation. Lobular CA is characterized by a high incidence of multicentricity and bilaterality as well as Indian file histology. Paget's disease of the breast is an underlying ductal CA w/extension to the overlying nipple. Microscopically it is characterized by large cells w/ hyperchromatic nuclei and an abundant pale staining cytoplasm.

MALIGNANT BREAST TUMORS

D • Ductal (infiltrating ductal eg. scirrhous)

I • Inflammatory

M • Medullary

• Mucinous

P • Phyllodes = cytosarcoma

L • Lobular

E • Eczematous change w/Paget's disease of the breast

OVARIAN TUMORS

The following story is helpful for learning the classification system of ovarian tumors. Imagine that you have gone to the store and bought a basket containing **"EG(G)S"** (eggs). You notice that there is a deed tag attached to the basket which shows proof of purchase. As you are leaving the store, the security guard questions your ownership of the basket. Your reply is, "are you trying to **BSME, C** (see) **DEED TAG**". The first mnemonic describes the three catagories of ovarian tumors, epithelial, germ cell and sex cord stromal. The second mnemonic is a list of the tumors within those categories.

Epithelial

B • Brenner
S • Serous
M • Mucinous
E • Endometrioid

Germ Cell

C • Choriocarcinoma
D • Dysgerminoma
E • Endodermal sinus tumor
E • Embryonal carcinoma
D • Dermoid cyst

Sex-Cord Stromal

T • Thecoma & fibroma
A • Arrhenoblastoma
G • Granulosa cell tumor

Staging of Cervical Cancer

The mnemonic for the staging of cervical cancer is "**CVPA**". This mnemonic is simplified to facilitate learning and retention. With experience, one can learn the staging system in more detail.

Stage

I.	**C**	→	Cervix
II.	**CV**	→	Cervix and Vagina
III.	**CVP**	→	Cervix, Vagina and Pelvic sidewall
IV.	**CVPA**	→	Cervix, Vagina, Pelvic sidewall and Adjacent organs

RISK FACTORS FOR ASCAD

Atherosclerotic coronary artery disease is the number one cause of death in the U.S.A. via CHF, MI and sudden death. A pt with all of these risk factors is a "**SAD BET**" to avoid the development of severe atherosclerosis. However, DM, HTN, elevated cholesterol and smoking are modifiable with medical Tx and pt cooperation. Therefore you should check every adult pt for the associated risk factors.

S • Sex = male

A • Age = middle age to elderly

D • DM

B • BP ↑

E • Elevated cholesterol

T • Tobacco

Family history is also an important risk factor.

ANGINA

Angina pectoris (AP) is chest discomfort/chest pain (CD/CP) due to transient myocardial ischemia that is usually caused by atherosclerotic lesions in the coronary arteries which make them unable to effectively respond to conditions of ↑ myocardial oxygen demand. CD on exertion is the most important clinical feature of angina. This CD typically lasts 1-10 minutes and is relieved by rest or nitroglycerin (NTG). CD lasting longer than 30 minutes is suggestive of a myocardial infarction.

AP can be classified into 4 groups: stable, unstable, Prinzmetal's and syndrome x. This can be remembered by the mnemonic, "**SUPER X**". Stable AP is most common and is characterized by a stable pattern of CD on exertion. CD is often described by pt's as a tightness, squeezing or pressure sensation. The CD may radiate to the left arm or other areas, eg. the neck, jaw or right arm.

Unstable AP may occur at rest as well as w/exertion. It is characterized by CD episodes of ↑ frequency, duration or severity. In comparison to stable AP, unstable AP is a more dangerous condition because it may immediately precede myocardial infarction. There are some subsets of unstable AP that have been referred to by other names such as crescendo angina and preinfarction angina. Pt's presenting w/an unstable pattern of CD should be admitted to the hospital for further diagnostic workup (eg. rule out MI) and more intensive management.

Prinzmetal's (variant) AP results from coronary artery vasospasm and usually occurs at rest, eg. in the early morning hours. The hallmark of Prinzmetal's AP is ST-segment elevation during episodes of ischemic CD. Calcium channel blockers are an important aspect of Tx for Prinzmetal's angina. Some pt's w/CD characteristic of ischemic origin have normal coronary arteriograms and an EKG that is not consistent w/Prinzmetal's AP. This presentation is called syndrome X and is thought to be due to microvascular disease undetectable by conventional coronary arteriograms. Tx options for these different types of AP include nitrates, Beta-blockers, calcium channel blockers, aspirin, PTCA and CABG.

S • Stable → occurs w/exertion

U • Unstable → occurs w/exertion or at rest, a/w ↑ freq. severity or duration

P • Prinzmetal's (variant) → usually occurs at rest, a/w ST-seg ↑, during episodes of CD

E • Exertional CD

R • Relieved by rest or NTG

X • syndrome X

Heart Murmurs *ANK

The timing of left sided valvular heart murmurs can be remembered by the mnemonic, "**(H)ARD ASS MRS MSD**".

(H)ARD	•	Aortic Regurgitaion	→ Diastolic
ASS	•	Aortic Stenosis	→ Systolic
MRS	•	Mitral Regurgitation	→ Systolic
MSD	•	Mitral Stenosis	→ Diastolic

CONGENITAL HEART DISEASE

CHD can be classified into three groups, left to right shunts, obstructive lesions and cyanotic lesions. In most cases the etiology is unkown. Risk factors include maternal CHD, alcoholism, lithium and Rubella infection. Down's syndrome (a/w septal defects), Turner's syndrome (a/w coarc of Ao) and several other congenital disorders are a/w increased incidence of CHD, and these can be remembered by the mnemonic, "**LOT**" which stands for **L**eft to right shunts, **O**bstructive lesions and **T5** (5 cyanotic lesions that start w/the letter T).

L • L to R shunt

1. VSD • most common CHD, Small are asymp & often close spont, large w/ ↑ shunt
2. ASD • 3 types = ostium primum, ostium secundum & sinus venosus
3. PDA • Tx = indomethacin or Surg

O • Obstructive lesions

1. Coarc Ao • usually just distal to left Subclavian artery, a/w UE HTN, ↓ femoral pulses
2. Ao Sten • eg. w/congenital bicuspid valve
3. Pul Sten • a/w dyspnea, fatigue, RVH

CONGENITAL HEART DISEASE

T • T_5 = Cyanotic lesions

1. TGA • survival requires ASD, VSD or PDA, CXR w/egg shape Ht, ↑ mixing w/Rashkind balloon atrial septostomy &/or Mustard operation

2. TOF • Pul st, overrd Ao, VSD, RVH, CXR w/boot shape Ht

3. TAPVR • Supracardiac, Cardiac, Infracardiac, CXR w/snowman/figure "8" Ht

4. Tricuspid atresia • a/w ASD, EKG w/LAD

5. Truncus arteriosus • single trunk exits from Ht

TETRALOGY OF FALLOT *ANK

The tetrad of cardiac abnormalities found in tetralogy of Fallot can be remembered by the mnemonic, "**POSH**".

P • Pulmonary stenosis

O • Overriding aorta

S • Septal Defect → VSD

H • Hypertrophy of right ventricle

NEPHROTIC SYNDROME

Nephrotic Syndrome (NS) is characterized by hypoalbuminemia, proteinuria and lipidemia. Important complications include protein malnutrition, hypercoaguable state and ↑ bacterial infections. These features can be remembered by the phrase Nephrotic "**NAPLES**". Minimal change disease is the most common cause of NS in children. Membranous glomerulonephritis is the most common cause of NS in adults.

N • NS

A • Albumin ↓

P • Proteinuria

L • Lipidemia

E • Edema

S • Sequelae/complications

→ 1. Protein malnutrition

2. Hypercoaguable state

3. ↑ bacterial infections

HEMATURIA *ANK

The most common causes of hematuria can be remembered by the mnemonic,"**SHIT**".

S • Stones

H • Hemoglobinopathy

I • Infection,

Intrinsic kidney disease,

Iatrogenic (eg. w/foley)

T • Tumors,

Trauma,

Toxins

CYSTITIS AND PYELONEPHRITIS

Bacterial infection of the bladder (cystitis) and the kidneys (pyelonephritis) is a very common medical problem. UTI's are more common in females, and in pt's w/the following risk factors, Diabetes mellitus, Reflux, Instrumentation, Pregnancy and Stasis (eg. 2° to obstruction). These can be remembered by the mnemonic, "**DRIPS**".

Urinary frequency, urgency and dysuria are common symptoms of cystitis. Urinalysis may reveal ↑ WBC (pyuria) and bacteriuria. Urine gram stain and culture are used to identify the microorganism. E. coli is the most common pathogen. Urine culture is considered positive when there are $>10^5$ CFU/ml. However, under certain conditions, smaller numbers are considered significant. The additional presence of fever, flank pain (CVA tenderness) and WBC casts in the urine are indicative of pyelonephritis.

D • Diabetes mellitus

R • Reflux

I • Instrumentation (eg. w/Foley catheter)

P • Pregnancy

S • Stasis eg. BPH, neurogenic bladder

RENAL PAPILLARY NECROSIS

The renal papillae look like little pads as they project into the minor calyces from which urine drains into the major calyces, then the renal pelvis and then the ureter. The predisposing factors for papillary necrosis can be remembered by the mnemonic, "**PADS**".

P • Pyelonephritis

A • Analgesic abuse

D • Diabetes mellitus

S • Sickle cell anemia

TESTICULAR TUMORS

Testicular tumors are most common in the 20 to 40 year old age group. Early diagnosis is very important because many testicular tumors respond well to treatment if found early. The typical presentation is a unilateral, firm, painless testicular enlargement.

Seminomas are the most common tumor, and usually have a good prognosis. The different types of testicular tumors can be remembered by the phrase "**Testis SETCIS**". Some testicular tumors produce AFP and/or HCG. Malignant testicular tumors tend to metastasize along the cord structures to the para-aortic lymph nodes. Pt's w/cryptorchidism have an increased incidence of testicular tumors.

S • Seminoma - most common, prognosis is usually good, radiosensitive

E • Embroynal

T • Teratoma

C • Choriocarcinoma - highly malignant, poor prognosis, ↑ HCG

I • Interstitial (Leydig) cell - usually benign

S • Sertoli cell - usually benign

Lupus

SLE is one of the most common and most terrible autoimmune diseases. Feared by both the layman and the physician, it was the central focus of the recent movie "Gross Anatomy." Many of us know, or know of persons afflicted with SLE.

When one of your patients has ANA ⊕ and the criteria for Dx are also ⊕. You might say to yourself oh "SHIT," she's got SLE. The short form of the mnemonic is **$(SH_2I_2T_2)_3$** because 3 items are associated with each letter.

S •	Skin	1. Malar & discoid rash
		2. Oral & nasophar ulceration
		3. Photosensitivity
H •	Ht	1. Pericarditis & Pleuritis
		2. Myocarditis, MI & CVA
		3. Endocarditis, Libman -Sacks
H •	Hemo	1. ↓ plt
		2. ↓ WBC
		3. ↓ RBC

LUPUS

I	•	Imm	1. ANA
			2. dsDNA
			3. Sm
I	•	Imm	1. Histone with proc, hydral, INH
			2. VDRL positive
			3. LE cells & ↓ C3
T	•	Type III HS	1. Glomerulonephritis
			2. Arthritis
			3. Vasculitis
T	•	Tx	1. ASA & NSAID's & Antimalarials
			2. Steroids → Topical & Systemic
			3. Cytotoxic agents → azathioprine, cytoxan

PM/DM

Polymyositis (PM) is an inflammatory myopathy which causes proximal symmetric weakness of the UE & LE. For example, these pt's have difficulty rising from a chair, combing their hair or stepping onto a **MED-VAN**. Polymyositis when a/w a rash is called Dermatomyositis (DM).

M
- Myositis, prox symm myopathy
- Muscle biopsy ⊕

E
- EMG ⊕ w/fibrillations
- ENZ ↑ - ↑ CPK, Aldolase & Urinary Myoglobin

D
- Difficulty arising from chair, combing hair, stepping onto bus/ MED-VAN
- Dysphagia - ↑ risk aspiration

V
- Violaceous heliotrope rash of eyelids
- Variable presentation, eg. DM especially common if a child is affected

A
- AutoAb - PM & Jo
- Abnormal moa relative to most autoimm diseases - b/c it's cell mediated

N
- Neoplasm - ↑ risk of malig - eg. lung CA
- N - kNuckles w/MP rash = Gottron's Sx

MULTIPLE ENDOCRINE ADENOMATOSIS

Multiple Endocrine Adenomatosis (MEA) type I is characterized by Pituitary tumors, hyper-Parathyroidism and Pancreatic tumors. This can be remembered by the phrase, "**Pit-Para-Panc**". MEA type II is associated with hyper-Parathyroidism, Medullary carcinoma of the thyroid and pheochromocytoma which often arises from the adrenal Medulla. This can be remembered by the phrase, "**Para-Medullary-Medulla**".

Type I MEA → **Pit-Para-Panc**

Type II MEA → **Para-Medullary-Medulla**

THE ANEMIAS

The anemias can be classified into 3 groups based on cell size, microcytic, macrocytic and normocytic. The anemia's in these categories can be remembered by the mnemonic, **LITA'S-BARF-IN HIS CHART**.

MICRO

L • Lead- ped pt's w/pica, a/w basophilic stippling of RBC's

I • IDA - most common anemia ↓ Ferritin, ↑ TIBC

T • Thalassemia

A • ACD - ↓ Fe rel from RES, ↓ TIBC, Ferritin WNL or ↑

S • Sideroblastic - blk heme syn - Fe in Mito - encircles Nuc=Ringed Sideroblast

MACRO

B • B12 ↓ - eg. lack IF/Pern Anemia

A • Alcohol

R • Reticulocytes ↑

F • Folate ↓ - eg. ↓ intake, hypersegmented polys

THE ANEMIAS

N/N

I • Inf - eg. Malaria, hepatitis

N • Nocturnal - eg.PNH

H • Hb disorders - eg. HbSS

I • IEM

S • Shape abn - 1. spherocytes

2. Stomato

3. Ellipto

4. Acantho

C • Chemical eg. Aldomet, Sulfonamides

H • Hypersplenism

A • AutoAB - eg. Warm (IgG), Cold (IgM), HDN, Transfusion RXN

R • Renal dis - CRF, HUS

T • TTP & other causes Trauma to RBC eg. prosthetic Ht valves microangiopath hemolytic anemia

RBC Inclusions

In certain physiologic and pathologic conditions, RBC's have inclusions. These can serve as useful diagnostic findings. This mnemonic can be remembered by the phrase, "RBC's can have almost as many inclusions as herbal **(H_2IRBal)** tea."

H • Howell - Jolly bodies

→ composed of DNA/nuclear framgents, eg. post splenectomy states

H • Heinz bodies

→ composed of ppt denatured Hb, eg. w/G6PD deficiency

I • Iron = pappenheimer bodies = siderocytes

R • Reticulocytes

→ composed of RNA, eg. w/hemolysis or after hemorrhage

B • Basophilic stippling

→ eg. w/lead poisoning

TTP

Thrombotic Thrombocytopenic purpura is an acute onset systemic disease that is most often seen in young adult-to-middle aged pt's. The characteristic pentad of symptoms is thrombocytopenic purpura, fever, anemia, neurologic signs and symptoms (S & S), and renal failure. These can be remembered by the mnemonic, "**T2ANK**". The pathogenesis appears to be the formation of widespread platelet microthrombi that lodge in the small arterioles and capillaries causing microangiopathic hemolytic anemia, as well as damage to the brain and kidney. Currently, plasmapheresis along with other supportive measures is regarded as the Tx of choice.

T • TTP

T • Temperature ↑

A • Anemia

N • Neurologic S & S

K • Kidney dysfunction/renal failure

POLYCYTHEMIA VERA

Polycythemia vera is a neoplastic proliferation of marrow stem cells. The typical pt is elderly or late middle age and c/o ruddy (plethoric) complexion, headaches (HA), dizziness and pruritis. Their is also ↑ risk of occlusive/thrombotic episodes eg. cerebrovascular, coronary or venous. Secondary transformation to myelofibrosis or acute leukemia may occur.

In the presence of the above mentioned clinical features, further w/u is used to confirm the Dx of polycythemia vera. Dx requires the presence of three major criteria or the first two major criteria and any two minor criteria. The major criteria are ↑ ↑ RBC, normal O_2 saturation and splenomegaly. The minor criteria are elevated plt's, WBC, LAP and Vitamin B12. Polycythemia vera is Tx by phlebotomy which may be supplemented by radioactive phosphorus or chemotherapy. The clinical features and diagnostic criteria of polycythemia vera can be remembered by the mnemonic, "**ROSE**".

	Clinical Features	Diagnostic Criteria
R	• Ruddy (plethoric) complexion, HA, dizziness, pruritis	• RBC ↑ ↑
O	• Occlusive/thrombotic episodes	• O_2 sat = normal
S	• Secondary transformation to myelofibrosis or leukemia may occur	• Spleen ↑
E	• Elderly and late middle age pt's	• Elevated plt's, WBC, LAP, Vitamin B_{12}

Multiple Myeloma

MM is a malignant proliferation of plasma cells. The typical pt is an elderly person presenting w/back pain and anemia. Serum electrophoresis shows monoclonal elevation of an immunoglobin eg. IgG or IgA. Urine electrophoresis may demonstrate the presence of light chains (Bence - Jones protein).

Other useful lab findings may include ↑ ESR, rouleaux formation, ↑ Tp/albumin ratio, ↑ Ca^{2+} and proteinuria. This protein will ppt if the urine is heated, i.e. if you "**BAKE IT**". Bone x-rays may show osteolytic lesions of the axial skeleton with associated osteoporosis. The definitive Dx of MM is made by detection of >10% plasma cells in a bone marrow aspirate.

As the disease progresses pt's may develop polyradiculopathy 2° to compression fractures of the vertebrae, renal failure and severe infections. Tx includes chemotherapy (CT), radiotherapy (RT) of some bone lesions and symptomatic Tx of other complications eg. ↑ Ca^{2+}, infections and anemia.

B • Bone

→ 1. most common 1° malig bone tumor

2. bone pain/back pain/radiculopathy 2° to osteolytic lesions

3. marrow aspirate > 10% plasma cells

MULTIPLE MYELOMA

A • Anemia

→ 1. Anemia

2. ↑ Tp/Alb, gamma spike on SPE, ESR ↑, rouleaux

K • Kidney

→ 1. Renal failure 2° to ↑ Ca^{2+}, Lt. chains, amyloid

2. Renal failure is 2nd most common cause of death

E • Elderly

→ Elderly pt's

I • Infection

→ 1. most common cause of death

2. ↓ functional Ig → ↑ infections eg. Strep pneumoniae

T • Tx

→ CT, RT pneumococcal vaccine & symptomatic Tx of complications

WISKOTT- ALDRICH SYNDROME

Wiskott-Aldrich syndrome is an X-linked disease that presents in infancy with eczema, petechiae and recurrent infections. The recurrent infections are due to an inability to produce antibody to polysacchride antigens. These pt's have ↑ IgA and ↑ IgE levels, but ↓ IgM. The characteristic manifestations of Wiskott-Aldrich syndrome can be remembered by the mnemonic, "**WATER$_X$-CHOMP**". There is also an ↑ incidence of malignancies of the reticuloendothelial system. The Tx of choice is marrow transplant.

W • Wiskott-Aldrich syndrome

A • IgA ↑

T • Thrombocytopenia → petechiae

E • Eczema & IgE ↑

R • Recurrent infections

X • X-linked

CHO • CHO = carbohydrate = difficulty w/polysacchride antigens

M • IgM ↓
• Malignancies ↑
• Marrow transplant = Tx of choice

P • Platelets are small in size

OBSTRUCTIVE LUNG DISEASE

The most important types of obstructive lung disease can be remembered by the mnemonic, "**BABE**". Chronic bronchitis and emphysema often occur in combination. Consequently, these two diseases are often grouped together under the term COPD (Chronic Obstructive Pulmonary Disease).

B • Bronchiectasis

A • Asthma

B • Bronchitis, chronic

E • Emphysema

Kartagener's Syndrome

Kartagener's syndrome is characterised by the triad of bronchiectasis, sinusitis and situs inversus. In addition there is an ↑ incidence of otitis media (OM). These pt's have chronic respiratory infections and immotile spermatozoa due to a defect in the dynein arms of the microtubule axoneme in cilia. Kartagener's syndrome is a subset of the immotile cilia syndome which can occur in the absence of situs inversus. The clinical features of Kartagener's syndrome can be remembered by the mnemonic, "**BOSSI**".

B • Bronchiectasis

O • OM

S • Sinusitis

S • Situs inversus

I • Infertility

PLUMMER VINSON SYNDROME

PVS is rare in the U.S.A., but relatively common in Scandinavia and Great Britain. The typical pt is a middle aged female w/atrophic glossitis, dysphagia and IDA. The upper esophageal web can be demonstrated by endoscopy or barium swallow. The characteristic features of this condition can be remembered by the phrase, "**Plummer's Little WEDGE**". Pt's usually respond well to Tx w/Fe supplementation and endoscopic dilation/rupture of the esophageal web.

Plummer's = PVS

Little = microcytic, hypochromic anemia = IDA

W • Women of middle age

E • Esophageal web

D • Dysphagia

G • Glossitis (atrophic) & angular stomatitis

E • Endoscopic dilatation/rupt. of webs and Fe supplement is usually an effective Tx.

"BARRIER BREAKERS"

The following drugs are either directly or indirectly harmful to the gastric or duodenal mucosa, and in general should be avoided in pt's w/peptic ulcer disease (PUD). These barrier breakers can be remembered by the mnemonic, "**CASA**". This mnemonic can also be used to ↑ compliance in pt's w/PUD by helping them to remember to avoid caffeine, aspirin, smoking and alcohol.

C • Caffeine

A • Aspirin, NSAID's

S • Smoking, Steriods

A • Alcohol

ACUTE PANCREATITIS (I)

The most common causes of acute pancreatitis are alcohol abuse and gallstones. There are many other less common etiologies. The causes of acute pancreatitis can be remembered by the mnemonic, "**ABCD-LIST**".

A • Alcohol

B • Biliary disease (eg. gallstones)

C • Calcium ↑ & Cancer of pancreas

D • Drugs

L • Lipids ↑

I • Infection (eg. mumps)

S • Surgery post-op

T • Trauma

ACUTE PANCREATITIS (II)

The clinical findings in acute pancreatitis can be remembered by the mnemonic, "**PANCITIS**". Pt's usually present w/abdominal pain as well as nausea and vomiting (N/V). In addition to the tender abdomen, PEx may show Turner's Sx, Cullen's Sx and manifestations of hypotension or shock, which occurs 2° to excessive loss of fluid into the peritoneal cavity. Therefore, fluid replacement is a very important aspect of Tx.

Laboratory examination may reveal ↑ amylase, ↑ lipase, ↑WBC and ↓ calcium. X-rays may demonstrate pleural effusion and Ileus. Tx includes fluid replacement, NPO, nasogastric suction, analgesics and symptomatic Tx of complications.

P • Pulmonary → pleural effusion

A • Abdominal → pain = epigastric radiates to back

N • N/V

C • Calcium ↓, amylase ↑, lipase ↑, WBC ↑

I • Ileus

T • Turner's Sx & Cullen's Sx

I • IVF (fluid replacement = v. important aspect of Tx)

S • Shock

CHRONIC PANCREATITIS

Chronic pancreatitis results from permanent structural damage to the pancreas, usually 2° to alcohol abuse in adults. In children chronic pancreatitis may occur 2° to cystic fibrosis. The characteristic features may be remembered by the mnemonic, "**SAD PAIN**". Due to exocrine deficiency pt's may develop malabsorption and steatorrhea. Due to endocrine deficiency pt's may develop diabetes mellitus. The pain is often continuous, and intractable pain is the main indication for surgery. Abdominal x-ray shows pancreatic calcifications and ERCP may demonstrate "chain-of-lakes" appearance due to ductal dilation. Fibrosis w/in the head of the pancreas may lead to common bile duct obstruction and the development of jaundice. Tx includes analgesia, replacement therapy (eg. pancreatic enzymes and insulin) and symptomatic Tx for other complications eg. surgery for ductal obstruction or intractable pain.

S • Steatorrhea/malabsorption

A • Alcohol associated

D • Diabetes

P • Pain

A • Abd XR w/calcifications

I • Icterus ±

N • Normal amylase

JAUNDICE

The list for causes of jaundice is "**HUGE**".

H • Hemolysis

U • Uptake ↓

G • Glucuronyl transferase ↓

E • Excretion

• Extrahepatic obstruction

CIRRHOSIS

The mnemonic for the causes of cirrhosis is "**CEBAH3**".

C • Cirrhosis

E • EtOH

B • Biliary

A • Alpha - 1- antitrypsin deficiency

H • Hemochromatosis
• Hepatolenticular degeneration (= Wilson's disease)
• Hepatitis

HBV Serology

The antigens and antibodies of HBV serology can be remembered by the phrase, "**feces SECES**".

S → HBsAg

E → HBeAg

C → HBcAb

E → HbeAb

S → HbsAb

MALIGNANT BONE TUMORS

A useful way to remember the most common malignant bone tumors is by making a list of their 1st initials eg. "**M-E-O-G-C-M**". The first M represents metastatic tumors which are the most common malignant tumor found in the bone. The other neoplasms are 1° tumors of bone and are listed in approximate chronological order according to the ages at which they occur. The pt's age and the location of the tumor are helpful features for DDx.

M • Metastatic

E • Ewing's sarcoma

O • Osteogenic sarcoma

G • Giant cell tumor

C • Chondrosarcoma

M • Multiple myeloma

NEUROCUTANEOUS SYNDROMES

The neurocutaneous syndromes (phakomatoses) are a group of diseases characterized by lesions of the nervous system and skin. These neurocutaneous diseases can be remembered by the mnemonic "**V_2AST**".

V • Von Recklinghausen's disease = neurofibromatosis

• Von Hippel-Lindau disease = retinocerebellar angiomatosis

A • Ataxia - telangiectasia

S • Sturge-Weber syndrome

T • Tuberous sclerosis

Chapter 5
Microbiology Synopsis

MICROBIOLOGY SYNOPSIS

CONTENTS

Introduction

"Microbiology synopsis" is designed to provide you with a concise systematic overview of clinical microbiology. It is a distillation of the most important information from classroom lectures, clinical experience, major textbooks, question books, practice tests and laboratory assignments. Its user friendly outline format quickly gives you the big picture and facilitates rapid review. By adding your own supplemental notes into the margin space, it becomes an ideal set of permanent condensed notes that will help you to prepare for in house exams and national boards part I.

There are two fundamental concepts that should be kept in mind when studying microbiology. The first is classification. You have to understand how microorganisms are classified, i.e. bacteria, fungi, viruses and parasites. Then within each of these groups there is further subclassification, eg. the bacteria group is made up of gram positives, gram negatives, mycobacteria, spirochetes and so on. The section on classification of DNA and RNA viruses employs several mnemonics which have been found especially helpful by students. By studying the table of contents and blocked out headings in each section of "Microbiology Synopsis" you can rapidly learn these classification systems.

The second fundamental concept is word association. When it comes to learning about individual microorganisms, less is more. It is more important to know several key facts about each microorganism than to try to learn a bunch of esoteric, nonclinical details that are ubiquitously found in big microbiology textbooks. For testing and clinical purposes you only need to know a few key associations for each microorganism. "Microbiology Synopsis" provides these key associations as well as a framework of classification so that you can rapidly learn the essentials of clinical microbiology.

BACTERIA

GRAM ⊕ COCCI

I. *Staphylococcus aureus*

Diseases	Comments
1. skin infections eg. carbuncles, furuncles, boils	1. catalase ⊕
2. osteomyelitis	2. coagulase ⊕
3. gastroenteritis/food poisoning	3. ferments mannitol
4. toxic shock syndrome	4. beta-hemolytic
5. endocarditis	5. golden yellow colonies
6. pneumonia	6. Protein A binds Fc portion of IgG
7. abcesses	7. most are pencillin resistant
8. scalded skin syndrome	

II. *Staphylococcus epidermidis*

1. endocarditis eg. w/prosthetic valves	1. catalase ⊕
	2. white colonies
	3. common skin flora

III. *Staphylococcus saprophyticus*

1. UTI	1. catalase ⊕
	2. Novobiocin resistant

GRAM ⊕ COCCI

I. *Streptococcus pyogenes*

	Diseases	Comments
1. **P**	• Pharyngitis	1. group A strep
2. **I**	• Impetigo	2. beta-hemolytic
3. **E**	• Erysipelas	3. bacitracin sensitive
4. **C**	• Cellulitis	4. streptolysin O
5. **E**	• Erythrogenic toxin → scarlet fever	5. streptolysin S
6. **S**	• Sequelae → rheumatic fever & poststreptococcal glomerulonephritis	

II. *Streptococcus agalactiae*

Diseases	Comments
1. neonatal sepsis	1. group B strep (GBS)
2. neonatal meningitis	2. beta-hemolytic
	3. CAMP ⊕
	4. hippurate hydrolysis

III. *Streptococcus faecalis* (*enterococcus*)

1. UTI
2. endocarditis

1. group D strep
2. growth in 6.5% NaCl
3. bile esculin hydrolysis

GRAM ⊕ COCCI

IV. *Streptococcus viridans* (eg. *Strep mutans*)

1. dental caries	1. oral flora
2. endocarditis	2. alpha hemolysis

V. *Streptococcus pneumoniae* (*pneumococcus*)

Disease/Comments

1. **C** • Conjunctivitis
2. **O** • Otitis
3. **M** • Media
4. **M** • Meningitis
5. **O** • Optochin sensitivity
6. **N** • Nasal sinusitis and ferments iNulin
7. **P** • Penicillin = drug of choice
8. **L** • Lobar pneumonia
9. **A** • Alpha hemolysis (= "green hemolysis")
10. **C** • Capsule → positive quellung reaction
11. **E** • Elderly persons are candidates for vaccination

GRAM ⊖ COCCI

I. *Neisseria gonorrhea*

Diseases	Comments
1. neonatal conjunctivitis	1. gram ⊖ diplococci
2. gonorrhea	2. oxidase ⊕
3. PID	3. ferments glucose N.g. → "g" for "g"lucose
	4. pili faciltate adherence

II. *Neisseria meningitidis*

Diseases	Comments
1. meningitis	1. gram ⊖ diplococci
2. Waterhouse -Friderichsen syndrome	2. oxidase ⊕
	3. ferments maltose & glucose N.m. → "m" for "m"altose

Gram ⊕ Rods

I. *Corynebacterium diptheriae*

Disease/Comments

1. **M** • Myocarditis
2. • Myelin degeneration
3. • Metachromatic granules
4. **A** • ADP ribosylating toxin
5. **P** • Pseudomembranous
6. **P** • Pharyngitis
7. **S** • Schick test

II. *Listeria monocytogenes*

1. listeriosis
2. neonatal meningitis

1. tumbling motility
2. growth at 4° C

III. *Erisypelothrix rhusiopathiae*

1. Erysipeloid skin lesions = painful, erythematous, edematous lesions of the skin, that are most often acquired from handling dead animal matter.

IV. *Actinomyces israelii*

1. actinomycosis	1. anaerobic
2. lumpy jaw	2. sulfur granules
3. PID in pt's w/IUD's	3. oral flora

GRAM ⊕ RODS - AEROBIC SPOREFORMERS

I. *Bacillus cereus*

Disease	Comments
1. Food poisioning eg. with reheated fried rice	1. aerobic 2. sporeformer

II. *Bacillus anthracis*

Disease	Comments
1. cutaneous anthrax	1. aerobic
2. pulmonary anthrax (woolsorter's disease)	2. sporeformer 3. polypeptide capsule

GRAM ⊕ RODS - ANAEROBIC SPOREFORMERS

I. *Clostridium difficile*

1. antibiotic associated pseudomembranous colitis

1. anaerobic sporeformer
2. Tx = Vancomycin "Vancomycin Vanquishes the difficult C. difficile"

II. *Clostridium perfringens*

1. gas gangrene
2. food poisoning

1. anaerobic sporeformer
2. double zone hemolysis
3. lecithinase, collagenase and hyaluronidase exotoxins

III. *Clostridium tetani*

1. tetanus

1. anaerobic sporeformer
2. "tennis racquet" appearance due to spherical, terminal spores
3. immunization = tetanus toxoid → requires booster
4. exotoxin = tetanospasmin

IV. *Clostridium botulinum*

1. botulism

1. anaerobic sporeformer
2. toxin inhibits ACh release

MYCOBACTERIA

I. *Mycobacterium tuberculosis*

1. classic pulmonary tuberculosis

1. acid fast rod
2. cell wall with high lipid content
3. Niacin ⊕
4. obligate aerobe
5. cord factor a/w virulence
6. intracellular growth in host
7. rough-buff colonies on Lowenstein-Jensen medium
8. grows slowly
9. PPD skin test
10. Tx includes INH Rifampin & PZA

II. *M. bovis*

1. intestinal tuberculosis eg. from unpasteurized milk	1. acid fast rod
	2. attenuated M. bovis used for BCG vaccine

III. *M. leprae*

1. leprosy	1. acid fast rod
	2. Tx includes dapsone

ATYPICAL MYCOBACTERIA

I. *Mycobacterium avium - intracellulare*

1. pulmonary infection in immunocompromised (IC) pt's eg. w/AIDS

II. *M. fortuitum*

1. pulmonary infection in IC pt's	1. rapid grower

III. *M. scrofulaceae*

1. Cervical lymphadenitis	1. scotochromogen

IV. *M. marinum*

1. cutaneous lesions eg. acquired from contact with contaminated water	1. photochromogen

V. *M. kansasii*

1. Pulmonary infection in IC host	1. photochromogen

GRAM ⊖ RODS - GI TRACT PATHOGENS

I. *Escherichia coli*

1. neonatal meningitis	1. gram ⊖ rod
2. UTI	2. facultative anaerobe
3. travelers diarrhea eg. entertoxigenic and enteroinvasive	3. IMVIC test = ++ - -
	4. ferments lactose
	5. EMB agar colonies with green metallic sheen
	6. H,O,K antigens a/w flagella, lipopolysaccharide & capsule

II. *Salmonella typhi*

1. typhoid fever

1. Lactose ⊖
2. H_2S^+
3. motile
4. variable flagella antigen
5. isolated from blood (early) and stool (late)
6. Carrier state may occur eg. w/gallbladder as resevoir of infection

GRAM ⊖ RODS - GI TRACT PATHOGENS

III. *Salmonella cholerasius*

1. septicemia

IV. *Salmonella enteritidis*

1. food poisoning/gastroenteritis

V. *Shigella spp.* (eg. *dysenteriae* & *sonnei*)

1. bacillary dysentery

1. Lactose ⊖
2. H_2S ⊖
3. non-motile

GRAM ⊖ RODS - GI TRACT PATHOGENS

VI. *Yersinia enterocolitica*

1. gastroenteritis with regional lymphadenopathy that mimics appendicitis

VII. *Bacteroides melanogenicus*

1. mixed anerobic infections
   eg. lung abcess

1. strict anaerobe
2. brown to black colonies
3. oral flora

VIII. *Bacteroides fragilis*

1. Complications of surgery
   eg. postoperative peritonitis

1. strict anaerobe
2. capsule a/w virulence
3. most common bacterium of normal bowel flora

GRAM ⊖ RODS - GI TRACT PATHOGENS

IX. *Vibrio cholerae*

1. Cholera	1. gram ⊖ curved rod
	2. oxidase ⊕
	3. grows well in alkaline pH
	4. toxin activates adenlylate cyclase leading to hypersecretion of electrolytes and water.

X. *Vibrio parahemolyticus*

1. gastroenteritis	1. gram ⊖ curved rod
	2. halophile
	3. kanagawa ⊕ strains
	4. acquired from improperly cooked, contaminated seafood

XI. *Vibrio vulnificus*

1. skin lesions	1. gram ⊖ curved rod
2. septicemia	2. halophile

XIII. *Campylobacter jejuni*

1. inflammatory diarrhea	1. gram ⊖ curved rod
	2. must be cultured under microaerophilic ($\downarrow O_2$) and capnophilic ($\uparrow CO_2$) conditions

GRAM ⊖ RODS - HAEMOPHILUS & BORDETELLA

I. *Haemophilus influenzae*

1. epiglottitis	1. pleomorphic gram ⊖ rod
2. meningitis	2. requires growth factors V (NAD) and X (hematin)
3. respiratory infections	3. satellite phenomenon
	4. polysaccharide capsule eg. type b

II. *Haemophilus ducreyi*

1. chancroid	1. gram ⊖ rod
	2. sexually transmitted
	3. causes soft, painful lesion

III. *Haemophilus aegyptius*

1. conjunctivitis ('pink eye')	1. gram ⊖ rod

IV. *Bordetella pertussis*

1. whooping cough (pertussis)

1. gram ⊖ rod
2. requires special media →Bordet-Gengou agar
3. pili facilitate adherence
4. encapsulated
5. causes lymphocytosis
6. whooping cough with three phases → catarrhal, paroxysmal and convalescent.

Gram ⊖ Rods - Pseudomonas & Moraxella

I. *Pseudomonas aeruginosa*

1. infections of wounds and burns
2. sepsis
3. catheter related UTI
4. nosocomial respiratory infections
5. infection of the eye

1. gram ⊖ rod
2. produces blue-green (pyocyanin-fluorescein) pigment
3. nonfermenter
4. exotoxin blocks elongation factor-II of protein synthesis
5. resistant to many antibiotics
6. may contaminate improperly maintained respiratory equipment

II. *Pseudomonas pseudomallei*

1. meliodosis

1. gram ⊖ rod

III. *Moraxella spp.* (eg. *lacunata*)

1. conjunctivitis	1. pleomorphic gram ⊖ rod 2. nonfermenter

GRAM ⊖ RODS - LEGIONELLA, KLEBSIELLA, SERRATIA & PROTEUS

I. *Legionella pneumophila*

1. legionnaire's disease (pneumonia)	1. gram ⊖ rod
2. pontiac fever	2. can grow in an aquatic environment eg. air conditioners
	3. Tx includes erythromycin

II. *Klebsiella pneumoniae*

1. lobar pneumonia	1. gram ⊖ rod
2. UTI	2. encapsulated

III. *Serratia Marcescens*

1. UTI	1. gram ⊖ rod
	2. resistant to many antibiotics

IV. *Proteus spp* (eg. *mirabilis & vulgaris*)

1. UTI
2. renal calculi

1. gram ⊖ rod
2. highly motile
3. swarming on solid media
4. urease ⊕

ZOONOSES

I. *Brucella spp* (eg. *suis*, *melitensis*, *abortus*)

1. brucellosis (eg. with undulant fever)

1. gram ⊖ coccobacillus
2. multiplies intracellularly
3. transmitted by unpasteurized milk or handling infected animal tissue

II. *Yersinia pestis*

1. bubonic plague
2. pneumonic plague

1. pleomorphic gram ⊖ rod
2. bipolar staining
3. bubonic plague transmitted by rat flea
4. pneumonic plague transmitted by respiratory droplets

III. *Pasteurella multocida*

1. localized wound infection from cat bites & dog bites

1. gram ⊖ coccobacillus

IV. *Francisella tularensis*

1. tularemia

1. pleomorphic gram ⊖ rod
2. highly virulent
3. transmitted by handling infected rabbits or from the bite of deerflies or ticks.
4. ulceroglandular is the most common type of tularemia.

Miscellaneous Bacteria

I. *Nocardia asteroides*

1. Opportunistic pulmonary infection	1. gram ⊕ 2. acid fast bacillus

II. *Eikenella corrodens*

1. Wound infection from human bites (eg. "clenched fist injuries")	1. gram ⊖ rod 2. oral flora

III. *Gardnerella Vaginalis*

1. Nonspecific vaginitis	1. gram ⊖ rod 2. clue cells 3. Tx includes metronidazole

IV. *Calymmatobacterium granulomatis*

1. Granuloma inguinale 2. Donovan bodies	1. gram ⊖

SPIROCHETES

I. *Treponema pallidum*

1. syphilis	1. spirochete
1° → indurated, painless chancre	2. darkfield microscopy
	3. motility via axial filaments
2° → skin rash & lymphadenopathy	4. nonspecific test → RPR & VDRL
3° → gummas, neurosyphilis & aortic arch aneurysm	5. specific test → FTA-Abs
	6. penicillin = drug of choice

II. *Treponema pertenue*

1. yaws	1. spirochete
	2. seen primarily in children living in tropical regions

III. *Treponema carateum*

1. pinta	1. spirochete

IV. *Leptospira interrogans*

1. Leptospirosis (eg. w/fever & jaundice)	1. spirochete 2. often shaped like a "question mark" 3. transmitted by contact w/water contaminated by infected animal urine

V. *Borrelia recurrentis*

1. relapsing fever	1. large spirochetes visible w/light microscopy 2. transmitted by louse or tick bite 3. recurrent spikes of fever appears due to antigenic variation

VI. *Borrelia burgdorferi*

1. Lyme disease

1. spirochete
2. transmitted by tick bite
3. Lyme disease a/w skin rash called erythema chronicum migrans

MYCOPLASMA & UREAPLASMA

I. *Mycoplasma pneumoniae*

1. primary atypical pneumonia ("walking" pneumonia)

1. lacks cell walls
2. requires sterols for growth
3. smallest bacteria to be cultured on cell free media
4. colonies w/"fried egg" appearance
5. atypical pneumonia w/non-productive cough
6. chest X-ray often suggests more significant infection than indicated by physical findings
7. cold agglutinins

II. *Ureaplasma urealyticum*

1. nongonococcal urethritis (NGU) in men

1. lacks cell walls
2. urease ⊕
3. formerly called T-strain (Tiny) mycoplasma

RICKETTSIAL DISEASES

I. *Rickettsia rickettsia*

1. Rocky Mountain Spotted fever (RMSF)	1. gram ⊖ 2. obligate intracellular parasite 3. vector = dog tick & wood tick 4. vasculitis/endothelial damage 5. Weil-Felix reaction for Ox-19 & Ox-2 6. Tx includes tetracycline

II. *R. akari*

1. rickettsial pox	1. vector = house mouse mites 2. characteristic lesion is black eschar

III. *R. Prowazekii*

1. Epidemic (louse borne) typhus	1. vector = lice
2. Brill's disease	

RICKETTSIAL DISEASES

IV. *R. typhi*

1. Endemic (murine) typhus	1. vector = fleas

V. *R. tsutsugamuchi*

1. Scrub typhus	1. vector = mites

VI. *Coxiella burnetii*

1. Q fever	1. acquired by inhalation of contaminated aerosols 2. There is no arthropod vector & Q fever occurs without a rash

CHLAMYDIAL DISEASES

I. *Chlamydia trachomatis*

Diseases	Characteristics
1. inclusion conjunctivitis	1. gram ⊖
2. trachoma	2. obligate intracellular parasite
3. lymphogranuloma venereum	3. cannot make ATP
4. nongonococcal urethritis (NGU)	4. basophilic cytoplasmic inclusion bodies
5. PID	
6. neonatal conjunctivitis	
7. neonatal pneumonia	

II. *Chlamydia psittaci*

Diseases	Characteristics
1. Psittacosis (ornithosis)	1. gram ⊖
	2. obligate intracellular parasite
	3. acquired from infected poultry (eg. turkeys) pet psittacines (eg. parrots & parakeets)

FUNGI

DERMATOPHYTES

Dermatophyte infections occur in the keratinized areas of the skin, hair & nails. These infections are usually self limited. Dermatophytes are classified into three genera, Microsporum, Epidermophyton and Trichophyton. Examples of dermatophyte infections are listed below. The diagnosis is made by examination of skin scrapings placed in KOH. Some dermatophytoses are also diagnosed by fluorescence under Wood's light. Dermatophytoses are Tx with topical antifungals, and oral griseofulvin is also given in more severe infections.

Three genera

I. **M** • *Microsporum*

II. **E** • *Epidermophyton*

III. **T** • *Trichophyton*

Dermatophytoses

1. *Tinea pedis* (athlete's foot)
2. *Tinea cruris* (jock itch)
3. *Tinea corporis* (ringworm)
4. *Tinea barbae*
5. *Tinea capitis*

YEASTS

I. *Candida albicans*

1. thrush	1. yeast
2. vulvovaginitis	2. reproduces by budding
3. opportunistic infections	3. pseudohyphae
	4. chlamydospores
	5. blastospores

II. *Cryptococcus neoformans*

1. meningitis	1. yeast
	2. reproduce by budding
	3. wide capsule
	4. india ink test
	5. latex agglutination test
	6. a/w pigeon droppings

FUNGAL DIMORPHS

I. *Sporothrix schenkii*

1. sporotrichosis (lymphocutaneous)	1. fungal dimorph
	2. yeast phase w/"cigar shaped" buds
	3. enters skin by traumatic inoculation

II. *Blastomyces dermatitidis*

1. pulmonary infection	1. fungal dimorph
2. cutaneous lesions	2. yeast phase with broad based buds

III. *Paracoccidioides brasiliensis*

1. pulmonary infection	1. fungal dimorph

FUNGAL DIMORPHS

IV. *Histoplasma capsulatum*

1. histoplasmosis (pulmonary infection)	1. fungal dimorph
	2. yeast phase located intracellularly
	3. mold phase with tuberculate chlamydospores

V. *Coccidioides immitis*

1. pulmonary infection (eg. San Joaquin Valley fever)	1. fungal dimorph
	2. yeast phase has spherule with endospores
	3. mold phase with arthrospores
	4. endemic to southwestern United States

VIRUSES

DNA VIRUSES

Viruses can be classified according to structure, site of replication & type of nucleic acid. The characteristic features of DNA viruses are double stranded DNA, nuclear replication, naked outer layer and icosahedral structure. The mnemonic for these characteristics of DNA viruses is, "**DN_2I**".

D • Double stranded DNA (ds DNA)

N • Nuclear replication

• Naked

I • Icosahedral

DNA VIRUSES - CLASSIFICATION *ANK

In general DNA viruses are naked, w/linear, dsDNA, Nuclear replication and icosahedral stucture. The exceptions are listed below. The DNA viruses can be remembered by the phrase, "DNA viruses are **H_2 A P P_2 (Y)*** families."

DNA viruses	naked	linear	ds DNA	N. repl	Icosa
H • Herpes	enveloped				
H • Hepadna	enveloped	circular			
A • Adeno					
P • Papova		circular			
P • Parvo			ss DNA		
P • Pox	complex			Cytopl	complex
(Y)					

DNA VIRUSES - DISEASES

Herpes

1. **HSV-1** → herpes labialis/cold sores, gingivostomatitis keratoconjunctivitis, encephalitis.

2. **HSV -2** → genital herpes, neonatal herpes

3. **EBV** → heterophile ⊕ infectious mononucleosis, Burkitt's lymphoma, nasopharyngeal cancer

4. **CMV** → opportunistic infections, heterophile ⊖ infectious mononucleosis, congenital CMV

5. **V-Z** → Chickenpox
   Shingles

Hepadna

1. **HBV** → Hepatitis B, hepatocellular cancer

Adeno

1. **Adeno** → Pharyngoconjunctival fever, epidemic keratoconjunctivitis

DNA VIRUSES - DISEASES

Papo

1. **HPV** → cutaneous warts and genital warts
2. **Polyoma**
3. **SV40**
4. **JC** → PML
5. **BK**

Parvo

Pox

1. **Variola** → Smallpox
2. **Vaccinia** → used for vaccine to smallpox
3. **Molluscum contagiosum**
   → skin lesions

RNA VIRUSES

The characteristic features of RNA viruses are ssRNA, plus or minus, enveloped outer layer, cytoplasmic replication and helical structure. The mnemonic for these characteristics of RNA viruses is, "**S P E (E) C H**".

S • Single stranded RNA (ssRNA)

P • Plus or minus (⊕ or ⊖ RNA)

E • Envelope

(E)

C • Cytoplasmic replication

H • Helical

RNA VIRUSES - CLASSIFICATION

In general RNA viruses are enveloped with ssRNA, cytoplasmic replication and helical structure. The mnemonic for RNA viruses is derived from the author's name. His initials are PR, however, with important documents, such as those requiring carbon paper, he signs his full name which is represented by the initials PTR. The RNA viruses can be remembered by the mnemonic "**PR- CARBO(N)-PTR**".

RNA viruses	enveloped	ssRNA	Cyto repl	Helical
P • Paramyxo		⊖	Nuclear & Cyto	
R • Retro		⊕		
C • Corona				
A • Arena				
R • Rhabdo		⊖		
B • Buny				
O • Orthomyxo		⊖	Nuclear & Cyto	
(N)				
P • Pico	naked	⊕		Icosa
T • Toga		⊕		Icosa
R • Reo	naked	ds RNA		Icosa

RNA VIRUSES - DISEASES

Paramyxo

1. Parainfluenza
   → croup
2. Measles → measles
3. Mumps → mumps
4. RSV → bronchiolitis

Retro

1. HIV → AIDS
2. HTLV → adult T-cell leukemia
3. MMTV
4. ASV

Corona → common cold

Arena → LCM

Rhabdo → rabies

RNA VIRUSES - DISEASES

Buny → California encephalitis

Orthomyxo

1. Influenza → influenza

Pico

1. **P** • Polio → polio
2. **E** • Echo → enteritis and meningitis
3. **R** • Rhino → common cold
4. **C** • Coxsackie → herpangina, HFM-disease, myocarditis
5. **H** • HAV → hepatitis A

RNA VIRUSES - DISEASES

Toga

1. **A** • Alpha → VEE, EEE, WEE

2. **R** • Rubi → rubella

3. **F** • Flavi → St. Louis encephalitis, yellow fever, dengue

Reo

1. Rotavirus → infant diarrhea

2. Orbivirus → Colorado tick fever

PARASITES

For most of us, the thought of parasites brings to mind bad memories of memorizing bizarre lifecycles, a desire to wash one's hands again and all in all a bad case of the wilies.

However these creatures have worldwide medical importance, and a basic understanding of their classification system will make them much more manageable to learn. The key is to remember the parasitic **PART** of the phylogenetic tree. This mnemonic will trigger your memory to recall the parasite's scientific and clinical manifestations. **SAFCO** and **WHAT-PP-FLO** are just nonsense words to help you remember the protozoans and roundworms.

P • Protozoa
- **S** • Sporozoa
  - Malaria
  - Cryptosporidosis
- **A** • Ameba (E.h., N.f.)
- **F** • Flagellates
  - Giardia
  - Trichomonas
  - Trypanosomas
  - Leishmanias
- **C** • Ciliates (B. coli)

PARASITES

(O) • other

(A) • Arthropods

R • Roundworms (Nematodes)

W • Whip (T.t.)

H • Hook (N.a., A.d.)

A • Ascaris (A.l.)

T • Thread (S.s.)

P • Pin (E.v.)

P • Pork (T.s.)

F • Filiariasis (Elephantiasis)

L • Loiasis

O • Onochercha v.

PARASITES

T • Tapeworms (Cestodes)

1. Beef (T.s.)
2. Pork (T.s.)
3. Fish (D.l.)
4. Dog (E.g.)
5. Human (H.n.)

T • Trematodes

1. Blood flukes Schistosomas h.j.m.
2. Liver flukes F.h., C.s.
3. Lung fluke-P.w.

CHAPTER 6
M-3 MNEMONICS

INTERNAL MEDICINE MNEMONICS

HISTORY AND PHYSICAL EXAM

Every medical school has a course where students learn to obtain a medical history and perform the physical exam. The transition from classroom medicine to clinical medicine is difficult for all students. The following concepts will help ease the transition.

Use a mnemonic to learn/remember the format/framework of the history and physical exam (H & P). This is the essential clinical information which all complete H & P's should include. It is expected that you will add to it and make adjustments as suited to the individual pt. Use of a mnemonic facilitates an orderly systematic approach that will enhance your thoroughness. This is especially helpful when your beeper goes off in the middle of the night and you need to rapidly orient yourself. Also this orderly systematic approach will make it easier for others to read your H & P's.

Speaking of which, please write neatly. This is just common courtesy to the other people who will need to read your H & P. If your handwriting is illegible, then your notes are worthless. You might as well just urinate on the chart. Communication between health care professionals is one of the most important purposes of the H & P. A good H & P should concisely summarize the pertinent aspects of the pt's clinical situation in a way that facilitates development of a plan for Tx and further Dx w/u.

Equally important is the communication between you and your pt's. Conduct yourself in an organized, empathic, professional manner that will put the pt at ease. Periodically, summarize your understanding of what the pt has told you. This gives the pt a chance to correct errors and to supplement where necessary. At the end of the interview, allow time for the pt's questions. A useful guideline is to make sure that your pts are treated with the same consideration and thoughtfulness that you would want provided for members of your own family that were in a hospital.

The mnemonic for the Hx is "**CHAMP-For-SAT**". The mnemonic for the physical exam is "**GVH-NB-RHAP-ESR-NMS-MSE**". This sequence was chosen to facilitate anatomical continuity and economy of movement. Notice that the PEx works downward from head to toe. You can, of course, adjust the order as appropriate to the individual pt. Memorizing a format enables you to be flexible while keeping sight of your goals.

Hx

- **C** • CC
- **H** • HPI
- **A** • Allergies
- **M** • Meds
- **P** • PSH
  PMH
- **F** • FH
- **S** • SH
- **A** • Alcohol
- **T** • Tobacco
  IVDA
  Review of systems

HISTORY AND PHYSICAL EXAM

PEx

G • General

V • Vital signs

H • HEENT

N • Neck

B • Back

R • Respiratory

H • Heart

A • Abdomen

P • Peripheral Vascular

E • Extremities

S • Skin

R • Rectal
Reproductive

N • Neuro

M • Motor

S • Sensory

MSE • Mental Status Exam

EKG Interpretation

EKG carts are like battering Rams ("**R2HAMS**") when medical students are rushing to the room of a pt having chest pain. This mnemonic takes you step-by-step thru EKG interpretation. You should check for all of these things on every EKG you read: **R**ate, **R**hythm, **H**ypertrophy, **A**xis, **M**yocardial infarction (Q waves), **S**T-segments and T-waves. The section on rhythms is further subcategorized by the mnemonic, **SANDI-B** (pronounced SANDY-B) which represents **S**inus, **A**trial, **N**odal, and **D**eadly (= ventricular) rhythms as well as a reminder to check for abnormal **I**ntervals and conduction **B**locks. Follow the sequence of the mnemonic step-by-step and you will be amazed at how quickly and effectively you can interpret EKG's. You must read the EKG systematically. First scan the anterior leads, V_{1-4}. Then the lateral leads $V_{5, 6}$, AV_L, I. Then the inferior leads AV_F, II, III.

R • Rate = nl, brady, tach, 300-150-100-75-60-50

R • Rhythm =

- **S** • Sinus - NSR, Sinus brady, Sinus tach
- **A** • Atrial - Atrial tach, WAP, MAT, AFlut, AFib
- **N** • Nodal - Nodal Pm, accel Nodal Pm (nlQRS but without P-waves)
- **D** • Deadly (=Vent) - PVC's, VT, VFib

EKG INTERPRETATION

- **I** • Intervals - PR > .2 is AVB, QRS > .12 is BBB
- **B** • Blks - Sinus, AVB 1°, 2°, 3°, RBBB, LBBB
- **H** • Hypertrophy - LAE, RAE, RVH, LVH
- **A** • Axis - I^+ F^+ = nl, I^- F^+ = RAD, I^+ F, II, III^- = LAD
- **M** • MI - Q-waves - Ant w/$V_{1\text{-}4}$, LAT w/AV_L, I
  Inf w/F, II, III, Post w/large R and STdepr $V_{1,2}$
- **S** • ST - segments - indicates acute injury
  T-waves - indicates ischemia when inverted
  Tx effects - eg. Dig
  electrolytes - eg. ↑ K^+, ↓ K^+

Endocarditis

Rheumatic fever (RhF) and Congenital heart disease (CHD) are major predisposing factors for the development of infective endocarditis (IE). IE usually presents w/fever, new onset ht murmur and embolic phenomena. Dx is made by Hx, PEx, blood culture (Cx) and echo. In this mnemonic "K" is a "wildcard" that represents the letter "E". When the Dx is made early, Tx with ABx has a high cure rate for SBE (Subacute Bacterial Endocarditis).

MR. FRANK SPARCKS is a Univiversity of Illinois administrator who had RhF as a child and then developed IE several years ago. Fortunately he was Tx successfully and is now back at the U of I where he is beloved by all medical students.

M • Mitral valve dis eg. 2° to RhF = predispos

R • RhF & CHD = predispos

F • Fever & new murmur

R • Roth's spots in Retina

A • Ao valve dis eg. 2° to RhF or w/congen bicuspid AoValve = predispos

N • "N"odes = Osler's "Nodes" & Janeway lesions on hands & feet

K → E-Emboli → Emboli to K & Spl
Splinter hem in nailbeds
Petechiae of buccal mucosa & extremities

ENDOCARDITIS

S • SBE → eg. Strep viridans inf of prev damaged valves

P • PVE → eg. Staph epidermidis & aureus (early) or Strep viridans (late)

A • ABE → eg. IVDA w/Staph aureus inf of tricuspid valve

R • Repl of valve ind → 1 severe CHF
2 persistent bacteremia
3 emboli-major recurrent
4 Fungal

C • Cx of blood + >90%

K → E-Echo detects veg

S • Std proph->Dental & URT proc w/PCN, GI/GU proc w/Amp & Gent

ACUTE CHEST PAIN → 5 KILLERS

*DR.GUSTAVO ESPINOSA

In patients with acute chest pain it is important to quickly Dx and Tx the following five conditions, because a delay in recognition can be deadly. The mnemonic for the five most common life-threatening conditions with acute chest pain is "**MAPPE**".

M • MI

A • Aneurysmal dissection (thoracic aorta)

P • Pulmonary embolus

P • Pneumothorax

E • Esophageal rupture

CHF

CHF is the inability of the heart to pump enough blood to meet the metabolic demands of the body. Left HF is a/w dyspnea, orthopnea, PND, pulmonary edema and ventricular gallop (S3). Left HF is also the most common cause of right HF. Right HF is a/w JVD, hepatic congestion and pedal edema. CXR may show cardiomegaly and pulmonary edema.

CHF is a syndrome, not a Dx. It can be caused by CAD, MI, HTN, valvular disease, cardiomyopathy and other diseases. It is useful to try to determine the underlying etiology so that Tx can be more specifically directed.

Tx of CHF requires a "**TEAM**" effort between patient, dietician, nurse and MD. The Tx modalities listed below may be employed to a greater or lesser extent depending on the individual pt. Dir, Dig, Dil, avoidance of salt and restricted physical activity are the mainstays of outpt management. In addition to these, the remaining modes are primarily utilized for a hospitalized pt w/pulmonary edema.

T • Tx = Dir, Dig, Dil = Diuretic, Digitalis, vasoDilator

E • Elevate head,
check Electrolytes, CBC, EKG and CXR
Eliminate precipitating/aggravating factors

A • Airway (give O_2)
Adrenergic stimulants
Avoid salt

M • Minimal activity (eg. bedrest)
Monitor (eg. check vital signs frequently)
Morphine (causes venous dilation & ↓ pt anxiety)

DVT AND PE

The typical pt with a DVT or PE usually has some of the following risk factors, eg. elderly, overweight, post-op, trauma, CHF, or immobilized. Pt's with DVT and PE certainly do not resemble **A PACE HORSE**. PE is one of the most common causes of sudden death in hospitalized pt's. It is important to quickly Dx and Tx PE's because they are often recurrent, often lethal when recurrent and often preventable with adequate anticoagulation.

DVT

D •	Deep v thrombosis	**D**oppler
V •	Virchow's triad	**V**enogram
T •	Tenderness, swelling, Homan's$^+$	**T**x = anticoagulation

Risk Factors

- **P** • Preg
- **E** • Elderly, eg. with CHF
- **S** • Stasis, eg. post-op

DVT AND PE

- **N** • Neoplasia, eg. pancreatic CA
- **O** • Obesity, Ocp's with xs estrogen, Orthopedic pts
- **T** • Trauma

Dx

- **A** • Arteriogram, V/Q scan

- **P** • PEx- dyspnea, ↑ RR, ↑ HR, LGF & CP hemoptysis a/w infarct
- **A** • ABG - hypoxic, resp alkalosis - ↓ PO_2, ↓ Pco_2, ↑ pH
- **C** • Cxr - WNL or Westermark's Sx or wedged shape density a/w infarct
- **E** • Ekg - Tach, S_1 ST_2 Q_3 inverted T_3

Tx

- **H** • Heparin
- **O** • Oxygen, Oral anticoag
- **R** • Recanalize
- **S** • Surg → eg. Greenfield filter
- **E** • Embolectomy

HEMOPTYSIS

The mnemonic for causes of hemoptysis is "**$(BIC)_2$**".

	Common causes		Less common causes
B	• Bronchitis	**B**	• Bronchiectasis
I	• Infection (eg.TB)	**I**	• Infarct (eg. with PE)
C	• Cancer	**C**	• Cardiac (eg. mitral stenosis)

PLEURAL EFFUSION (I)

A pleural effusion is an abnormal accumulation of fluid in the pleural space. Pt's may present with dyspnea and pleuritic pain (a sharp, stabbing pain that is ↑ with deep inspiration and coughing). Physical examination reveals ↓ to absent breath sounds and dullness to percussion over the area of effusion.

Small effusions are more readily seen on the lateral CXR and will appear as blunting of the costophrenic angle. Larger effusions cause opacification of the lung fields with a concave meniscus (an upward) curved shadow towards the lateral chest wall. Subpulmonic effusions may be seen as pseudoelevation of a hemidiaphragm on upright films and fluid shift over the inferior chest wall on lateral decubitus films.

The next step in the differential diagnosis of a pleural effusion is the thoracocentesis. This fluid is sent to the lab for measurement of total protein, LDH, pH, glc, RBC and WBC. It is also sent for gram stain, AFB stain, culture and cytology to check for infection or malignancy.

It is useful for differential diagnosis to categorize effusions as transudative or exudative. A transudative pleural effusion has a protein content less than 3g/dl and a pleural fluid vs. serum protein ratio less than .5, as well as an LDH content less than 200 and pl fluid to serum LDH ratio less than .6. The most common transudative effusions are caused by CHF, cirrhosis, nephrotic syndrome and starvation. The mnemonic, "**CHAMPS**" is helpful for working towards the DDx of a pleural effusion. Exudative effusions have ↑ amounts of protein and LDH. The most common exudative pleural effusions are pneumonia, TB and malignancy. Tx is directed towards the underlying cause and is also adjusted according to the severity of symptoms and whether or not the effusion is recurrent.

Pleural Effusion (II)

C • CHF
Cirrhosis (with ascites)
Chylothorax

H • Hemothorax (eg. with trauma)
Hepatic infection (with upward spread)
Hypothyroidism

A • AFB⊕
Asbestos
Albumin ↓ (with nephrotic syndrome and starvation)

M • Malignant 1°
Malignant 2°
Meig's syndrome

P • Pneumonia
Pulmonary embolism (with infarction)
Pancreatitis

S • SLE (or rheumatoid arthritis)
Saline overload
Side effect of drugs

UGIB

The most common causes of Upper GastroIntestinal Bleeding can be remembered by the mnemonic, "**PIETO**".

P • PUD → Duodenal & Gastric

I • Itis → Gastritis

E • Esophageal varices

T • Tears → Mallory-Weiss tear

O • Other → (eg. Gastric CA)

Lower GI Bleed

Don't be a chump. In a pt. with suspected LGIB you must R/O an UGIB source. The most common causes of LGIB can be remembered by the mnemonic, "**DA-CHUMP**".

D • Diverticulosis

A • Angiodysplasia

C • Colitis (eg. ulcerative colitis)

H • Hemorrhoid

U • UGIB

M • Malignancy

P • Polyp

HEPATIC ENCEPHALOPATHY

Hepatic encephalopathy is a neurologic syndrome that may accompany advanced liver disease. It is characterized by mood changes, confusion, disorientation, asterixis, drowsiness, stupor and coma. Ammonia levels in the blood are elevated. An important part of Tx is the recognition and removal of precipitating (ppt) factors. The mnemonic for the ppt/aggravating factors of hepatic encephalopathy is "**PACKINGS**". Dietary protein restriction, lactulose and neomycin are also important aspects of Tx.

P • Protein ↑ (dietary)

A • Alkalosis

C • Constipation
Contracted volume (=volume depletion)

K • K^+ ↓

I • Infection

N • Nitrogenous cpds ↑ in blood is a/w hepatic encephalopathy

G • GIB (gastrointestinal bleed)

S • Sedatives

GLUCAGONOMA

Glucagonoma is an alpha-cell tumor of the pancreas. Pt's develop a characteristic syndrome of clinical features that can be remembered by the mnemonic "**DAN'S Glucagonoma**". Serum glucagon levels are elevated.

D • Diabetes

A • Anemia

N • Necrolytic migratory erythema

S • Stomatitis

Glucagonoma → ↑ glucagon levels

NORMAL PRESSURE HYDROCEPHALUS *ANK

The classic triad of normal pressure hydrocephalus (NPH) can be remembered by the "**3-W's**".

W • Wet → incontinence

W • Wobbly → ataxia

W • Wacky → dementia

FELTY'S SYNDROME

FS is occasionally seen in pt's w/chronic seropositive RA. The characteristic features of FS can be remembered by the phrase Felty's "**FAULTS**". This includes leg ulcers, ↓ PMN's, ↓ plt's and splenomegaly. In Felty's syndrome the spleen is often felt. The ↓ PMN's leads to ↑ susceptibility to infections. Pt's w/recurrent infections or significant morbidity due to other hematological abnormalities, usually benefit from Tx w/splenectomy.

F • FS

A • Arthritis = chronic RA

U • Ulcers of leg

L • Leukopenia/neutropenia = ↓ PMN's

T • Thrombocytopenia

S • Splenomegaly

REITER'S SYNDROME

The classic presentation is a young male with a recent Hx of **U**rethritis who develops **S**kin symptoms, **A**rthritis and **C**onjunctivitis. This disease can also follow an episode of **D**ysentery. A small percentage of pts develop **C**arditis with aortic insufficiency. The features of Reiter's syndrome can be remembered by the mnemonic, **USA-CDC**.

U • Urethritis

S • Skin KB - Keratoderma Blennorrhagicum
CB - Circinate Balanitis

A • Arthritis

C • Conjunctivitis

D • Dysentery

C • Carditis - w/aortic insufficiency

SURGERY MNEMONICS

PREOPERATIVE NOTE

The pre-op note should be written the night before surgery. It should include the Dx, planned procedure, labs, EKG and CXR. It should also confirm that blood is available in the blood bank if necessary, that the pre-op orders have been written and that the consent has been signed.

Although the format will vary somewhat depending on the type of procedure and the age of the pt, the following outline is a useful guideline. The format of a typical pre-op note can be remembered by the mnemonic, **P_2-SALE-BOC** pronounced (P_2-SALE-BOCK).

P • Preoperative Dx

P • Planned procedure

S • Surgeon

A • Allergies

L • Labs eg. electrolytes, CBC, UA, PT/PTT

E • EKG & CXR

B • Blood

O • Orders

C • Consent

POST-OP NOTE

The format of the post-op note can be remembered by the mnemonic, **P_3-SAFE-DCFS_2**.

P • Pre-op Dx

P • Post-op Dx

P • Procedure

S • Surgeons

A • Anesthesia

F • Fluids

E • Estimated blood loss (EBL)

D • Drains

C • Complications

F • Findings

S • Specimens

• Status eg. transferred to RR in stable condition

POST-OP ORDERS *ANK

A • Admit

D • Dx → S/P surg procedure for disease

C • Cond

V • VS

A • Activity

• Allergies

N • Nsg → eg. strict I/O's, daily wt's

D • Diet → eg. NPO

• Drains → eg. JP to bulb sxn, foley to gravity, record output q8°

I • IVF → eg. D5 1/2 NS with 20 meq KCL per liter @ 100 cc/hr

M • Meds → eg. pain meds, chronic meds, ABx

E • Extras

L • Labs → eg. CBC, SMA - 6

APPENDICITIS

Appendicitis is the most common condition requiring acute abdominal surgery. Obstruction, eg. by fecalith or lymphoid hypertrophy is the key factor in the development of appendicitis. The appendix continues to produce secretions distal to the obstruction, and this leads to distension which can further lead to bacterial overgrowth, increased luminal pressure, ischemia, infarction and perforation.

The classic presentation is pain and anorexia followed by vomitting (V). The pain is initially periumbilical and then over the course of several hours localizes to the right LQ. Right LQ pain is the most important symptom for making the Dx of appendicitis. Anorexia is a useful finding since it is almost always present with appendicitis. The sequence of symptoms has diagnostic significance with the usual order being anorexia and pain followed by V.

Physical findings are determined by the anatomic location of the appendix and by how far the disease has progressed. The presence of rebound tenderness indicates peritoneal irritation. Physical findings such as Rosving's sign, obturator sign and psoas sign can also be helpful for making the Dx.

The temperature elevation of appendicitis is usually mild and the leukocytosis moderate, eg. 10,000 - 17,000. Higher fevers or WBC may indicate a complication such as perforation. Perforation occurs more frequently in young children and in the elderly because the presentation is more likely to be atypical and the Dx delayed. They are also more likely to progress to peritonitis because of the immature omentum in young children and the atrophic omentum in the elderly. The Dx findings and potential complications of appendicitis can be remembered by the mnemonic **"PAVEL'S P's"** (P5).

APPENDICITIS

P • Pain

A • Anorexia

V • V

E • Elevated temperature

L • Leukocytosis

S • Sx's eg. rebound, Rosving's, obturator, & psoas

P • 1. Perforation

2. Phlegmon

3. Periappendiceal abcess

4. Peritonitis

5. Pyelthrombophlebitis

Intestinal Obstruction

Adhesions, hernias and tumors are the most common causes of intestinal obstruction in adults. The Dx is made by history and physical as well as X-rays. The characteristic findings of the history and physical can be remembered by the mnemonic "**CODE**".

C • Crampy abdominal pain

Constipation

O • Obstipation

Old abdominal scar

D • Distention

Dehydration

E • Emesis

• Empty vault

POSTOP FEVER *ANK

During your surgical rotation you will see many pt's with postop fevers. This mnemonic is very useful.

W • Wind → Atelectasis and pneumonia

W • Water → UTI

W • Walk → DVT/PE

W • Wound

W • Wanes → Veins → check IV site(s)

Acute Arterial Occlusion *ANK

The characteristic clinical features of acute arterial occlusion can be remembered by the **"6-P's"**.

P • Pain

P • Pallor

P • Pulselessness

P • Poikilothermia

P • Paralysis

P • Paresthesias

Tx of Intracranial Hypertension

The mnemonic for the treatment of increased intracranial pressure is "**Fluid Drainage HOSE**".

F • Furosemide

D • Drainage

H • Hyperventilation

O • Osmotic agents (eg. mannitol, glycerol)

S • Steroids

E • Elevate head

FRACTURE OF THE SCAPHOID

Fracture of the scaphoid is relatively common in young adults following a fall on an outstretched hand. Physical exam shows tenderness over the scaphoid in the anatomical snuffbox. Fractures of the scaphoid have a relatively high incidence of complications such as AVN, Nonunion and 2° DJD. The mnemonic for the clinical features of a fractured scaphoid is "**SANDY**". Initial x-rays are sometimes negative, eg. w/an undisplaced fracture of the scaphoid. If fracture is present x-rays will usually become positive w/in one to several weeks. Therefore in a young adult w/the above mentioned Hx and PEx, the fracture should be Tx/immobilized (eg. w/a plaster cast) and then x-rayed again at a later date.

S • Snuffbox tender

A • AVN

N • Nonunion

D • DJD

Y • Young adults

COLLE'S FRACTURE

Colles fracture occurs most commonly in adults over the age of 50 years, women more often than men. It is produced by falling onto an outstretched hand. The characteristic features of a Colles fracture can be remembered by the "**3-D's → D_1, D_2, D_3**".

- **D_1** • Distal radius fracture
- **D_2** • Dinner fork Deformity
- **D_3** • Dorsal Displacement of Distal fragment

DEQUERVAIN'S STENOSING TENOSYNOVITIS

The mnemonic for the characteristic features of DeQuervain's stenosing tensynovitis is "**FATE**".

- **F** • Finkelstein test
- **A** • APL → abductor pollicis longus tendon entrapment
- **T** • Tx = splinting, NSAID's, steroid injection & surgical release (when indicated)
- **E** • EPB → extensor pollicis brevis tendon entrapment

TUMORS METASTATIC TO BONE *DR. GUSTAVO ESPINOSA

The most common tumors metastatic to the bone can be rembered by the mnemonic, "**BLT's with Ketchup and Pickles**". Prostatic carcinoma is the most common cause of blastic metastases. The other tumors listed typically produce osteolytic metastases.

B • Breast

L • Lung

T • Thyroid

K • Kidney

P • Prostrate

OBSTETRICS/GYNECOLOGY

HYDATIFORM MOLE

The letter "**H**" in the word "H"ydatiform mole can be used to represent the characteristic features of the classic, complete hydatiform mole.

"H"ydatiform mole

1. "**H**"ydropic villi
2. "**H**"CG is ↑
3. "**H**"ypertension
4. "**H**"is chromosomes (paternal origin)
5. "**H**"er karyotype (XX)

ECTOPIC PREGNANCY *ANK

The mnemonic for ectopic pregnancy is **"AMP2ULLAR(Y)"**.

A • Abnormal vaginal bleeding

M • Missed menses

P • Pelvic pain
• Pregnancy test positive → determines pregnancy ⊕

U • Ultrasound → empty uterus → determines ectopic

L • Laparoscopy → determines location

L • Losing blood (eg. with ruptured ectopic)

A • Ampullary & isthmic = most common locations

R • Risk factors = PID, IUD, Endometriosis, previous ectopic

(Y)

CARDINAL MOVEMENTS OF LABOR & DELIVERY

The mnemonic for the seven cardinal movements of labor and delivery during childbirth is "**EDy FIE3**".

E • Engagement

D • Descent

F • Flexion

I • Internal rotation

E • Extension

• External rotation

• Expulsion

BREECH

The mnemonic for the different types of breech presentation is "**FIC**".

F • Frank

I • Incomplete

C • Complete

ABNORMAL UTERINE BLEEDING

The mnemonic for causes of abnormal uterine bleeding is "**PINES**".

P • Pregnancy disorders

I • Infection

N • Neoplasm

E • Endocrine disorders

S • Systemic conditions

PEDIATRIC MNEMONICS

REYE'S SYNDROME

Reye's syndrome is characterized by acute encephalopathy and liver dysfunction that occurs primarily in children following a recent viral illness, eg. w/varicella or influenza. Mitochondrial dysfunction is a key feature in the pathogenesis. Aspirin ingestion in a child w/a viral infection also appears to be a/w development of Reye's syndrome.

The typical pt has a h/o recent viral illness and then develops protracted vomiting (V) and lethargy. This may progress to confusion, combativeness and coma. If the pt's condition continues to decline, brainstem reflexes are lost, decerebrate rigidity is present and spontaneous ventilation is lost. The clinical features of Reye's syndrome can be remembered by the mnemonic, "$\mathbf{A_1\text{-}V_2\ C_3\ R_4}$".

These pts also usually have ↑ LFT's, ↑ ammonia, and ↑ PT/PTT. Ammonia levels greater than 300 are a/w poor prognosis. Tx is mostly supportive w/measures to control cerebral edema, respiratory failure, ↑ ammonia, ↑ PT/PTT and hypoglycemia. Fortunately, the prognosis has been greatly improved in recent years due to earlier diagnosis and intensive management.

REYE'S SYNDROME

A • Aspirin

V • Viral illness → (V) and lethargy

C • Confusion
Combativeness
Coma

R • Reflexes ⊕ (brainstem reflexes)
→ Reflexes ⊖
→ Rigidity (decerebrate)
→ Respiratory failure

SICKLE CELL ANEMIA

Sickle cell anemia is an important common disease. It occurs in approximately 1/500 American blacks. The molecular defect is the substitution of valine for glutamic acid in the sixth position of the B-globin chain. When deoxygenated, Hb S has ↓ solubility that causes the Hb S molecules to polymerize which distorts the RBC into a sickle shape. This sickling makes the RBC's more fragile which leads to chronic hemolytic anemia (HA). Sickling also makes the RBC's less flexible leading to trapping within the microcirculation and subsequent tissue infarction.

Pt's with sickle cell anemia start to develop symptoms at around 6 months of age as the HbF concentration becomes decreased. Avascular necrosis (AVN) of the marrow in the metacarpal and metatarsal bones leads to dactylitis (hand-foot syndrome). In infants, before splenic infarction has occurred, splenic sequestration may occur which can cause hypovolemic shock.

The spleen becomes non-functional at an early age and young children are highly susceptible to overwhelming infection with encapsulated bacteria eg. pneumococcus and H. influenzae. Therefore, penicillin prophylaxis and vaccination are an important aspect of preventive maintenance in sickle cell anemia.

Other type of crises include aplastic crises and vaso-occlusive crises. Aplastic crises occurs when viral infection leads to suppression of erythropoiesis in this pt who is already anemic. Vaso-occlusive crises are caused by occlusion of the microvasculature leading to extreme pain and to organ damage eg. aseptic necrosis of bones, CVA, Kidney damage, leg ulcers and other complications. Pt's with sickle cell anemia have an ↑ incidence of osteomyletis eg. with Staph aureus and Salmonella. Sickle cell nephropathy is characterized by ↓ urine concentrating ability, hematuria and papillary necrosis. The clinical features of sickle cell anemia can be remembered by the mnemonic, "**SICKLE PAD**".

The Dx of sickle cell anemia is suggested by the Hx and PEx as well as the presence of sickle cells on the peripheral smear. Definitive Dx is made by hemoglobin electrophoresis. Tx of sickle cell anemia includes preventive measures such as prophylactic penicillin, vaccination and avoidance of predisposing factors for vaso-occlusive episodes eg. dehydration, hypoxia and acidosis, as well as immediate Tx of infection and crises when they occur.

S • Sickle cell anemia
→ val for glu subst
→ ↓ sol w/ ↓ 0_2 sat → sickling → HA & tissue infarction

I • Infection
→ 1. fxn asplenics
2. Sepsis w/encap bacteria
3. Osteo w/Staph aureus & Salmonella

C • Crises
→ 1. Aplastic crises
2. Splenic sequestration
3. Vaso-occlusion

K • Kidney
→ ↓ urine conc ability, hematuria, papillary necrosis

L • Leg ulcers

E • Electrophoresis of Hb for Dx

SICKLE CELL ANEMIA

P • Preventive maintenance
→ prophylactic penicillin, vaccination
→ avoid ppt's for VO-crises

A • AVN eg. of femoral head

D • Dactylitis (hand-foot syndrome)

KAWASAKI'S DISEASE

Kawasaki's disease (and motorcycles) is an important "**FELLER**" of pediatric pt's. These letters represent the diagnostic criteria, i.e. **F**ever, conjunctivitis (**E**ye), oral inflammation (**L**ips and mouth), **L**ymphadenopathy, **E**xtremities involvement and a polymorphous **R**ash. The diagnosis is established when 5 of the 6 criteria are present.Thrombocytosis and coronary artery vasculitis w/ aneurysmal dilation are other important findings. Kawasaki's disease is Tx w/aspirin. Tx w/aspirin may be supplemented w/gamma-gobulin during the acute phase.

F • Fever ≥ 5 days

E • Eyes → bilateral conjunctival injection

L • Lips → cracked & dry
Tongue → strawberry appearance
Mouth → erythema of oropharynx

L • Lymphadenopathy → cervical

E • Extremities
Acute → erythema of palms & soles w/indurated edema
Subacute → desquamation beginning at fingertips
Convalescent → resolving

R • Rash → erythematous, polymorphous

CONGENITAL SYPHILIS

The characteristic lesions of congenital syphilis can be remembered by the mnemonic, "**SAN-TOBAS**".

S • Skin rash

A • Abortions ↑ & stillbirths ↑

N • Nose → saddle nose & snuffles

T • Teeth - Hutchinson's notched incisor, screwdriver teeth
- Mulberry molars w/extra cusps

O • Oral lesions

B • Bone lesions eg. osteochondritis, periostitis

A • Anemia

S • Saber shins

CONGENITAL TOXOPLASMOSIS

The mnemonic for congenital toxoplasmosis is "**THC3**". Toxoplasmosis infection can be congenital or acquired. The congenital form is associated with hydrocephalus, cerebral calcification and chorioretinitis. The acquired form in adults may present as a mononucleosis-like syndrome.

Congenital Toxoplasmosis

T • Toxoplasmosis

H • Hydrocephalus

C • Cerebral calcification

• Chorioretinitis

• Cat feces and raw meat are potential sources

VON HIPPEL-LINDAU SYNDROME

The mnemonic for Von Hippel-Lindau syndrome is "**CARR**".

C • Cerebellar hemangioblastoma

A • Autosomal dominant

R • Retinal hemangioma

R • Renal carcinoma

List of Mnemonics

PATHOLOGY

MICROBIOLOGY SYNOPSIS

INTERNAL MEDICINE

SURGERY

OBSTETRICS/GYNECOLOGY

PEDIATRICS

INDEX